# MASTER MANIPULATOR

# MASTER MANIPULATOR

## THE EXPLOSIVE TRUE STORY OF FRAUD, EMBEZZLEMENT, AND GOVERNMENT BETRAYAL AT THE CDC

### JAMES OTTAR GRUNDVIG

#### FOREWORD BY SHARYL ATTKISSON

#### INTRODUCTION BY ROBERT F. KENNEDY JR.

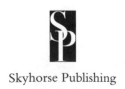

Skyhorse Publishing

Skyhorse Publishing books may be purchased in bulk at special discounts for sales promotion, corporate gifts, fund-raising, or educational purposes. Special editions can also be created to specifications. For details, contact the Special Sales Department, Skyhorse Publishing, 307 West 36th Street, 11th Floor, New York, NY 10018 or info@skyhorsepublishing.com.

Skyhorse® and Skyhorse Publishing® are registered trademarks of Skyhorse Publishing, Inc.®, a Delaware corporation."

Visit our website at www.skyhorsepublishing.com.
10 9 8 7 6 5 4
Library of Congress Cataloging-in-Publication Data is available on file.

Cover design: Rain Saukas
Cover photo: iStockphoto

ISBN: 978-1-5107-0843-3
Ebook ISBN: 978-1-5107-0844-0

Printed in the United States of America

# DEDICATION

to my son Fridrik
and his million brothers and sisters on the Autism Spectrum

# ACKNOWLEDGMENTS

This author wants to thank Louis Conte and Skyhorse Publisher Tony Lyons for providing the spark and resources, and for championing this book above and beyond the standard of such deeply researched projects. And for their continued support beyond the book's publication to uncover the truth, in all its stark reality, on a U.S. Department of Justice–indicted fugitive, who still today has not been extradited from his native Denmark to stand trial for his lead in the theft, money laundering, and racketeering crimes that diverted precious U.S. health grant money intended for autism research.

I would like to thank Danish journalists Jens Ramskov of *Engineering Magazine* and Peter Møller of Denmark's TV2 news station for their local research and professionalism. In the United States, I would like to thank the parents from all professional backgrounds in providing the insights, information, and research avenues to explore and drill down to the truth. They include my editor Michael Lewis at Skyhorse Publishing and Stephen Gregory the publisher of the *Epoch Times* newspaper, as well as Dr. F. Edward Yazbak, Helena Hjalmarsson, Mark Blaxill, Lyn Redwood, Sallie Bernard, Kim Mack Rosenberg, Robert Krakow, Dr. Brian Hooker, Dr. Andrew Wakefield, and Age of Autism editors Kim Stagliano and Dan Olmstead. In the United Kingdom, I want to thank John Dan Stone and David Thrower for their insights and years of research they have done on this most important issue.

And thanks to Fridrik's mother Lourdes Campos-Grundvig and to my late mother Gudrun Odfjell Grundvig for their support over the years.

I especially want to thank Robert F. Kennedy Jr. for his tireless support on one of the greatest stealth crises of our time, for bringing his energy, passion, and expertise to reverse a society-crippling epidemic, which as of the publication of this book marked 1 in 45 babies born in the United States acquired some form of Autism Spectrum Disorders. Mr. Kennedy has sacrificed a lot and given his all to the growing "autism community." He understands better than most that if we are capable of polluting the rivers, streams, land, air, and the oceans of the world, then we can environmentally contaminate infinitely smaller reservoirs and systems in babies, infants, and children before they have a chance to develop in the most crucial years of their healthy young lives.

Playing politics with the health of newborn babies is no longer an answer to solving and reversing the skyrocketing rates of children with autism. Not finding the root cause of the problem today will drain society of its resources and natural talent, while permanently removing future professionals from the labor force or ever becoming a productive member of this great nation.

# CONTENTS

# FOREWORD BY SHARYL ATTKISSON

Today fraudulent research and corruption are sadly becoming more commonplace. The case of Poul Thorsen, for example, stands out in terms of shameless audacity—stealing grant money meant for autism research. His actions only add to the questions of alleged corruption surrounding the Danish Studies designed to erase any association between vaccines and autism, sponsored by the world's premier public health agency: the Centers for Disease Control and Prevention (CDC).

One might expect fraud and corruption in government, but many Americans will be surprised to hear of it inside the CDC, the same agency that fumbled the arrival of Ebola virus on US shores in 2014. The fact that the CDC would contract with the likes of Dr. Thorsen on crucial research of vaccines and autism, and never consider setting aside his findings after his twenty-two-count criminal indictment, speaks to the waning credibility of the world's premiere public health agency.

# INTRODUCTION BY ROBERT F. KENNEDY JR.

Statistics don't lie, the saying goes, but statisticians do. As an environmental lawyer and veteran of hundreds of legal battles with some of the world's biggest polluters, I know that statistical—or epidemiological studies—are the go-to weapon of industry junk scientists. These hired guns—so called tobacco scientists—know that "fixing the science" or an epidemiological study is as easy as lighting up a smoke. For example, one could easily design an epidemiological study to "prove" that sex does not make one pregnant. The trick is simply to get rid of all the pregnant people before one analyzes the data. Now you have a study that shows lots of people having sex without consequence. Voila! That's one of the many tricks CDC's star biostitute, Poul Thorsen, used to deceive the public about the evidence linking mercury laced vaccines to autism. Prior to conducting his MMR study, Thorsen used "exclusions" to eliminate children with autism from the target population. Employing this and an inventory of other magician subterfuges, Thorsen authored a Danish study that CDC, for years, has been presenting as its gold standard evidence that thimerosal doesn't cause autism.

This is a story of how CDC used a con man to gull the public and ended up getting conned itself! Poul Thorsen is a world-class villain whose manipulation of health data gave CDC and big pharma what they wanted: a report clearing thimerosal of any possible role in the autism crisis. His story merits a book length expose because the fraud he casually helped orchestrate has had a monumental impact on the health of millions of children globally.

The Centers for Disease Control (CDC) most often cites Poul Thorsen's crooked research as the final word on the controversy linking vaccines to autism. CDC rarely mentions that Poul Thorsen is the subject of a twenty-two-count, 2011 indictment by the U.S. Department of Justice for wire fraud and money laundering in connection with more than $1 million in research grants that he pilfered from CDC while he ginned up fraudulent studies to "prove" that vaccines don't cause autism.[1] His crimes have won him a mug shot on the U.S. Department of Health and Human Services' (HHS) "most wanted" list.[2] Thorsen's former employer, Aarhus University—Denmark's university hospital system—permanently expelled him from practice in 2010. The fact that he is roaming free in Denmark and is easy to find, despite the federal indictment, indicates a lack of enthusiasm by HHS to file the necessary extradition papers and press for his capture. The agency has good reason to fear that a public trial would expose the pervasive corruption throughout CDC's vaccine division and the fragility of the science supporting CDC's claims about vaccine safety.

Dr. Thorsen is one of seven co-authors and the data manager for the two leading foreign studies offered by CDC as the foundation for its claims that vaccines do not cause autism. For nearly a decade, critics have pointed out that CDC's Danish studies are thinly veiled flimflam.[3] Besides employing the threadworm gimmick of

---

[1] "United States of America vs. Poul Thorsen" indictment, U.S. DOJ, April 13, 2011.

[2] https://oig.hhs.gov/fraud/fugitives/profiles.asp

[3] "Methodological Issues and Evidence of Malfeasance in Research Purporting to Show Thimerosal in Vaccines Is Safe," Brian Hooker et al., *BioMed Research International*, Vol. 2014.

manipulating exclusions to selectively eliminate kids, on some studies, with autism diagnoses from the study pool, Thorsen and his co-author used another novel dodge to "exculpate" mercury-laced vaccines. Thorsen's trick was not even a sophisticated brand of junk science, but it was a devastatingly effective way to deliver the conclusion CDC wanted. Thorsen's Madsen et al. 2003 ("Madsen 2003"),[4] purported to exonerate thimerosal—the mercury-based vaccine preservative— as the causative agent in the autism epidemic by showing that autism rates in Denmark increased after the Danish government removed thimerosal from vaccines in 1992.[5] But even the most casual critic could see that the increase in Danish autism was illusory since it was not actually based on an increased incidence of the disease. It was simply an artifact of Denmark's new reporting protocols.

Here's how Thorsen and his cronies pulled off this fraud: In 1993, the same year Denmark removed thimerosal-containing vaccines from distribution, it coincidentally required, for the first time, that outpatient autism cases be reported on the government's national disease registry. Prior to 1993, only inpatient cases were reported. These represented less than 10 percent of the total. Denmark's new reporting protocols increased the reported autism incidence cases by nearly 1300 percent. Dr. Thorsen and his pals took advantage of that artificial rise to suggest that real autism incidence had increased following thimerosal's ban. The authors also violated established peer-review scientific protocols by deleting the entire 2001-year class of seven-year-olds from the final published version.[6] That deletion was flagrant research

---

[4] "Thimerosal and the Occurrence of Autism: Negative Ecological Evidence From Danish Population-Based Data," Kreesten Madsen et al., *Pediatrics*, September 1, 2003.

[5] Dr. M. Hasse Letter to Commission of the European Communities, Committee for Proprietary Medicine Products, Re: "Organic Mercury Compounds as Antimicrobial Preservatives in Immunoglobulins," January 22, 1992.

[6] CDC internal email: "Application Tech Review" from Diana Schendel to Tom Horne, November 16, 2003.

fraud. The 2001 cohort was the first to be entirely free from thimerosal exposure in their vaccines. The subsequent analysis (Grønborg et al. 2013) of that data showed a steady decline in autism rates over a ten-year period following the removal of thimerosal in 1992.

Emails obtained under the Freedom of Information laws show that Thorsen, his co-authors, and CDC officials were all aware of these frauds when they published the study. Responsible journals, including *Lancet* and *JAMA*, rejected the Madsen study. It took a letter from the CDC's Jose Cordero, then director of its new National Center for Birth Defects and Developmental Disabilities (NCBDDD),[7] to strong-arm a lesser journal, *Pediatrics*, to finally publish the study. *Pediatrics* has earned notoriety as a frequent publisher of vaccine industry junk science. *Pediatrics* raises a substantial portion of its operating budget from vaccine makers. *Pediatrics* is the journal of the American Academy of Pediatrics, which is notorious for its conflicts with big donors. In 2016, the AAP was forced to drop its multi-million donor, Coca-Cola, as it's only "gold sponsor." In exchange for $3 million over six years, AAP had been shilling for the sugary drink maker, which it called a "distinguished" company due to Coke's commitment to "better the health of children worldwide." AAP only ended the mercenary romance when published exposes disclosed that Coke had been paying hired scientists to fix the science to "prove" that sugary drinks were not the culprit in the obesity epidemic.

At the 2007 National Academy of Sciences/Institute of Medicine (IOM) meeting, "Autism and the Environment: Challenges and Opportunity for Research," Dr. Irva Hertz-Picciotti, an internationally renowned environmental epidemiologist from the University of California, Davis, criticized the Madsen 2003 study for deliberately blurring outpatient and inpatient data sets: "The study, therefore is not a rigorous design, because you cannot compare the before and after

---

[7]   CDC Letter from NCBDDD Director Jose Cordero to Jerold F. Lucey, Editor-in-Chief Journal Pediatrics, December 10, 2002.

periods because of artifacts in how the database was constructed, and specifically how it changed over time." When CDC scientists finally took an authentic look at the Danish autism data a decade later, they demolished the conclusions in Madsen 2003. CDC's subsequent study, Grønborg et al. 2013, published in *JAMA Pediatrics*[8] directly contradicted Thorsen and Madsen. Grønborg and her co-authors found a 33 percent drop in autism spectrum disorder incidence in Denmark following the withdrawal of thimerosal in 1992.

Thorsen was also data manager for Kreesten Madsen's companion study on the MMR vaccine, Madsen et al 2002.[9] That study used similar deceptive statistical devices and flawed data to "prove" MMR safety.[10] That study employed CDC's trademark ruse of including many children who were too young to receive the autism diagnosis, which at that point usually occurred at age four in Denmark. CDC epidemiologists have consistently used this ploy in their phony autism research to dampen the autism signal in various studies. The 2002 Madsen MMR study also included a substantial number of unvaccinated children and employed a suite of other statistical gimmicks to mask the association with the MMR vaccine and dampen the autism signal.

Having trained in CDC's sophisticated fraud during his apprenticeship with the two notorious Madsen studies, it's no wonder that Poul Thorsen felt so at ease stealing more than $1 million that CDC had directed Thorsen to spend on managing data for those and other studies.

---

[8]  "Recurrence of Autism Spectrum Disorders in Full- and Half-Siblings and Trends Over Time A Population-Based Cohort Study," Therese K. Groenberg et al., *JAMA Pediatrics*, August 12, 2013.

[9]  "A Population-Based Study of Measles, Mumps, and Rubella Vaccination and Autism," Kreesten Madsen et al., *New England Journal of Medicine*, November 7, 2002.

[10]  "An Investigation of the Association Between MMR Vaccination and Autism in Denmark," G. S. Goldman and F. E. Yazbak, *Journal of American Physicians and Surgeons*, Vol. 9, Number 3, Fall 2004.

As James Grundvig brilliantly points out in the pages that follow, without Poul Thorsen, there would have been no Danish studies for the CDC to misuse all these years as the spear tip for its propaganda campaign on vaccine safety.

However, Grundvig gives us more; Thorsen was not a lone bad apple. Grundvig shows that CDC insiders, including Dr. Frank DeStefano (Director of the Immunization Safety Office); Dr. Marshalyn-Yeargin-Allsopp (Head of the Developmental Disabilities Branch); Dr. Diana Schendel, a CDC epidemiologist research scientist and Thorsen's longtime girlfriend, who in 2014 took a permanent position in the epidemiology department at Aarhus University, where Thorsen committed the theft of autism research money; and Dr. Coleen Boyle (Director of the National Center for Birth Defects and Developmental Disabilities) fully supported and orchestrated Thorsen's fraud. Boyle made her bones at CDC as lead investigator of 1984–1987 Congressional investigation of Agent Orange. In that post, Boyle and her team reported "no association" between the jungle defoliant dioxin and the grim inventory of rare cancers and autoimmune diseases that sickened tens of thousands of U.S. troops who fought in the war. Her work allowed the government to deny benefits and treatment for sickened soldiers for five years. In 1990, the Pentagon admitted during congressional hearings that Agent Orange was indeed the culprit. Today, Boyle is the director of CDC's National Center for Birth Defects and Developmental Disabilities. According to Dr. William Thompson, a seventeen-year CDC senior vaccine safety scientist and current CDC employee who recently filed for whistleblower status, Boyle and her team of researchers committed research fraud in a subsequent 2004 American study to conceal numbers suggesting that the MMR vaccine was associated with higher rates of autism in African-American children.

Poul Thorsen, the Master Manipulator, is the dark wizard of a federal agency that is steeped in corruption and compromised by financial entanglements with the pharmaceutical industry. Thorsen participated in a criminal conspiracy with his CDC bosses to distort science and fleece the American taxpayer. He then turned on his cronies and stole the money CDC paid him to conjure up his phony research. Thorsen's greatest crime, however, is the epidemic of millions of children with developmental disabilities who are the legacy of his fraud.

Dr. Poul Thorsen should be arrested and brought back to the United States to stand trial and receive justice. If that happens, we might see those in the CDC who sponsored his fraud be held finally accountable.

# PART I

# ERECTING THE MONOLITH

# THE BONE DEPOT OF ALUMINUM

Dr. John Clements suppressed the urge to sleep off the jetlag as he peered through the plate glass at the aquamarine inlet of El Borquerón—"wide opening"—watching the waves break against the rocks.

He had come a long way from Geneva, Switzerland, and longer still from the rolling green hills of his homeland in New South Wales, New Zealand, to attend the U.S. National Vaccine Program Office-sponsored workshop on aluminum in vaccines. The Caribe Hilton International Hotel in San Juan, Puerto Rico, was a major upgrade from the thimerosal workshop held the previous year in the sterile, 176-seat, Lister Hill Auditorium at the National Institutes of Health in Bethesda, Maryland. And for that he was thankful. Beyond being serene, the so-called 51st state of the United States was also far removed from the ravenous U.S. media and the prying eyes of the parents of autism spectrum disorder children. He knew the press blackout was only temporary, due to new freedom of information laws; one day the transcript on the aluminum workshop would get out. He understood that. But temporary would do for the success of the two-day conference since the August 1999 workshop on thimerosal had bordered on disaster. That summit drove a wedge of doubt into the U.S. vaccine program, suggesting more than a casual link that the mercury preservative in vaccines was the driving force behind the skyrocketing rates of autism in the United States. And solid scientists, like Dr. Clements, weren't fans of doubt.

The outdoorsman looked at the reflection of his hand in the window and gripped a fist, imagining he was holding his trusty walking cane. He saw himself on a ledge overlooking a Swiss valley and grasped the importance of the moment. Clements adjusted his wire-rimmed glasses and eyed the waves receding over the rocks before heading to the ballroom for the start of the "Workshop on Aluminum in Vaccines."

As the third speaker that morning, Dr. Clements, a 14-year medical officer of the Expanded Immunization Program with the World Health Organization in Geneva and previously New Zealand's Minister of Health, wouldn't be the one to inject doubt into the day's proceedings. He wondered if any of the leading experts on aluminum and immunizations would play the skeptic role and overturn a half-century of its use as an adjuvant in vaccines. Changing course on how vaccines were manufactured at the dawn of the new millennium would be akin to moving an alp to make room for a water park.

The costs, he calculated, would be staggering. It would require not only the search for a new adjuvant to replace the salts of aluminum hydroxide, aluminum sulfates, and aluminum phosphates, but years of clinical trials to prove that the new adjuvants would be safe, meeting both stringent U.S. Food and Drug Administration guidelines and U.S. Environmental Protection Agency standards.

Good luck with that, he thought as he ran the slides of his presentation, "Adjuvants in Vaccines—A Global Perspective," through his head for a final review.

To Clements's surprise, Dr. Martin Myers, the acting director of the National Vaccine Program Office, kicked off the proceedings by stating he would stand in for Dr. George Peter, the chairman of the National Vaccine Advisory Committee, because Peter couldn't get a plane out of Boston or Providence to fly to Puerto Rico on time.

Sans any humor, Marty Myers opened by saying, "Last summer we started a series of what we hope will be a series of symposia on the attitudes of vaccines. We talked about thimerosal last summer. We are talking about aluminum today and we plan to talk sequentially about each of the additives within vaccines."[11]

As the first speaker, an immunogenic expert from the University of Texas named Dr. Robert Hunter, discussed the use of adjuvants in vaccines, John Clements felt perspiration build up between his fingers. He wasn't nervous to speak, he just wasn't used to the humidity of the Caribbean.

Dr. Hunter held up a copy of the *Scientist*, and said, "I have here a copy of the *Scientist* newspaper that came out two weeks ago and the headline here is 'New Era in Vaccine Development.' The first sentence says, 'When all else fails, try something new.'"[12]

The audience laughed. But Dr. Clements knew that a new era in vaccines had begun, one in which it would become imperative for healthcare agencies and the pharmaceutical manufacturers to get out ahead of the story or risk losing the chance to immunize a 100 million children in the world from some of mankind's deadliest diseases. Add AIDS, Ebola, and Lyme disease to the dirty dozen that included TB, polio, and diphtheria toxoid, pertussis, and he knew the science of vaccines was locked in an arms race with mutating viruses and bacteria.

Perhaps that was what made Clements' hands sweat.

After an informal question and answer discussion with Dr. Hunter, Dr. Norman Baylor, the acting deputy director of the Office of Vaccine

---

[11] "Workshop on Aluminum in Vaccines," May 11, 2000 (page 1, lines 20–25) transcribed by Eberlin Reporting Services, Silver Springs, MD.

[12] Ibid (page 23, lines 5–9).

Research and Review and associate director for Regulatory Policy at Center for Biological Evaluation of Research at the Food and Drug Administration (FDA), took the podium.

Dr. Baylor presented "Aluminum Salts in Vaccines—A U.S. Perspective." He went on to list in a dry delivery the types of aluminum salts used as vaccine adjuvants. He was all business. Clements would expose that when he would speak next in a more natural, relaxed manner. Dr. Baylor then put his regulator's hat on and talked about U.S. Title 21, "Food and Drugs." Referring to part 610, "General Biological Products Standards," he said, "Now in the United States in the Code of Federal Regulations under 610.15, our 'Constituent Materials,' including preservatives and adjuvants, the amount of aluminum in the recommended individual dose of a biology product shall not exceed .85 milligrams of elemental aluminum."[13]

What Dr. Baylor left out from 610.15 was the main reason why the U.S. Health and Human Services (HHS) jointly sponsored the symposium with the Task Force for Child Survival and Development, a non-profit organization to improve the health of children worldwide—the safety of "biological" ingredients in vaccine products:

All ingredients used in a licensed product, and any diluent provided as an aid in the administration of the product, shall meet generally accepted standards of purity and quality. Any preservative used shall be sufficiently nontoxic so that the amount present in the recommended dose of the product will not be toxic to the recipient.[14]

"Purity and quality" of aluminum as a biological substance would be hard to come by, Dr. John Clements knew. As he watched Dr. Baylor

---

[13] Ibid (page 36, lines 7–12).

[14] http://www.accessdata.fda.gov/scripts/cdrh/cfdocs/cfcfr/CFRSearch. cfm?fr=610.15

fail to explain how the U.S. arrived at the "0.85 milligrams of aluminum per dose" standard and couldn't answer his question on why, during the late 1950s, the U.S. recommended using aluminum in vaccine adjuvants when the United Kingdom "backed away," Clements realized he needed his walking cane to lead the group in a new direction in a new age of immunizations. A message on safety would become just as critical as the effectiveness of and global reach for the childhood vaccine program.

On stage, Dr. Clements gave a broad smile and used his hiker's commanding view on the history of vaccines and adjuvants, leading up to the advancements made against other diseases, before touching upon the spotty "coverage" of vaccines with pregnant women. He noted the negative press on thimerosal. To allay the fears of new parents on vaccine safety, he said, "It is the mothers we are targeting and not infants."[15]

The WHO medical officer ran through the estimates on the number of neonatal (200,000) and maternal (30,000) deaths per year from tetanus alone and qualified those figures as being much higher. He went on to state the obvious—"There is no question that new vaccines equals the need for new adjuvants"[16]—before ascending to the heart of the matter of why there was the HHS second annual symposium on ingredients in vaccines for his next point.

"Secondly, just as thimerosal emerged its—can I call it—its ugly head last year and we were all thrown into a situation of siege momentarily until we got the facts out to the public, the public is very much interested in what is in vaccines and what their children are getting, and I believe this is something that we need to discuss in the next two days,"[17] Dr. Clements said, and added, "The public is very much concerned with mercury and it is not so surprising that thimerosal with its mercury generated so much interest. Aluminum is not perceived, I believe, by the

---

[15]  Ibid (page 59, lines 18–19).

[16]  Ibid (page 63, lines 24–25).

[17]  Ibid (page 64, lines 9–16).

public as a dangerous metal and, therefore, we are in a much more comfortable wicket in terms of defending its presence in vaccines."[18]

While not being a master orator, like most politicians, John Clements was a master tactician, and concluded by saying, "I think the public does have a right to know what is going on. I think the days of hidden administration are over and I do not think we should have any problem in disclosing what is in vaccines and what the risks are."[19]

The cold water on aluminum in vaccines came in the afternoon session. Pouring that water would be Sam Keith, PhD, an environmental health scientist with the Division of Toxicology at the Agency for Toxic Substances and Disease Registry (ATSDR). His presentation, "Toxicokinetics," discussed the harmful affects of skin penetrators, such as depleted uranium, the element used to harden military-grade shell casings in the Gulf War.

On adjuvants, he said,

> With aluminum, with it being injected by a syringe the situation is a bit more subtle. Be that as it may, aluminum, as uranium, is very prominent.
>
> Aluminum is the third most abundant element behind oxygen and silicon, which means it just happens to be in every media that humans enjoy in taking into their body. It is in the air we breathe. It is in the water we drink. It is in the food we eat.[20]

Dr. Keith worked his way through the presentation, laying out facts while not mincing words or minimizing the dangers aluminum can cause to the human body.

"But here is a critical one right here: 96 percent had been excreted through 1,178 days. And what does that mean? It means that there in

---

[18] Ibid (page 64, lines 17–24).
[19] Ibid (page 65, lines 5–9).
[20] Ibid (page 187, lines 10–18).

the body is a depot or 'that' is likely bone. But it also tells us that perhaps aluminum never reaches a steady state in the body, but accumulates over a number of years. That seems to be what we find as the human body tends to accumulate aluminum in the lung from almost nothing at birth to perhaps 20 to 30 milligrams at a ripe old age,"[21] he said, referring to a study done on the excretion of aluminum in rabbits and rats.

The first day's sessions concluded with a cocktail reception and dinner with an icy overhang ready to collapse on top of the U.S. vaccine program. And yet the tone had been set that messaging would be paramount to managing the growing public distrust in and the dampening of any backlash against metals used in vaccines. The resolve of getting that message out was made all the more urgent by Dr. Sam Keith's speech on aluminum as a toxic substance, a pole apart from the FDA's regulation ensuring that only ingredients with "purity and quality" make it into vaccines.

Prepared for such fallout, HHS lined up Dr. Max Lum, the director of Health Communications at the National Institute of Occupational Safety and Health, to wrap up the scientific session on day two, with his discussion "Communication Health Messages."

After highlighting his expertise as a "risk communicator" and the work he had done with the U.S. Surgeon General on the Gulf War, Dr. Lum embraced the message John Clements delivered, saying, "This is a new era. People are concerned. There is a high level of interest in health problems. The public acceptance in many cases depends on their participation and understanding and your personal credibility. Often, you are the message if you are delivering the particular message you have to deliver."[22]

Dr. Max Lum covered a lot of ground—from social media challenges and keeping the message positive to quoting old epidemiology

---

[21] Ibid (page 191, lines 10–24).

[22] "Workshop on Aluminum in Vaccines," May 12, 2000 (page 126, lines 14–21). transcribed by Eberlin Reporting Services, Silver Springs, MD.

studies to show a long track record on safety and calling a media-coined adverse reporting system at the CDC for what it was: a "secret database."

Max Lum concluded his motivational speech, asking, "How do we shape that message of hundreds of millions kids being protected against diseases?"[23]

Without a crystal ball showing the events that would transform the start of the 21st century—the 9/11 terrorist attacks, followed by two fronts on the war on terror, secret U.S. government doctrines, and the even more secretive "security state" of NSA sweeps of personal information of U.S. citizens—the need for transparency that John Clements espoused, and Dr. Max Lum alluded to, would all but disappear from the CDC.

The CDC would take control by setting a new course of shaping the message that thimerosal in vaccines was safe. It would start in three weeks in a secret meeting at the Simpsonwood retreat in Norcross, Georgia, where U.S. government agencies would comingle with big pharma industry leaders.

Sitting in the back, Dr. Robert Chen, chief of Vaccine Safety and Development for the CDC, took copious notes. He liked what Lum and Clements had to say but knew Simpsonwood would focus on the minutia of details and numbers-crunching of at least one major thimerosal study.

Although Dr. Clements was one of the fifty-two attendees invited to the Simpsonwood meeting, the CDC would begin its search to find someone to lead research studies that would disprove any links between vaccines and autism spectrum disorders.

That industry expert would need to play ball, be a foreigner, be known within the CDC circle of power, and work from a script a valley apart from the one Clements delivered on transparency. Masking data would be the key.

---

[23] Ibid May 12, 2000 (page 146, lines 10–11).

## 2

# DISOWNING THE FALLING STAR

On a cold, gray Friday morning on January 22, 2010, Jørgen Jørgensen, director of Aarhus University, Aarhus, Denmark, wondered what he had gotten himself into when he accepted the new position after having spent thirteen years as director at the exceedingly more sane and staid National Hospital. Stoic and not amused, the gray-haired fifty-three-year-old economist sat in his office reviewing the statement he had dictated, which had been reviewed internally by the university's board of directors and signed off by its lawyers and externally by the Danish Agency for Science, Technology and Innovation (DASTI).

Soon the two pages in Jørgensen's hand would be sent out as a press release. In effect, the statement would disown one of Aarhus's once rising stars in Dr. Poul Thorsen, a magnet and moneymaker for the university. All Jørgensen had to do was sign it and hand it to his assistant for distribution. Then all hell would break loose in the Danish newspapers, magazines, and social media channels, because a public flogging by a venerable institution of that kind was extremely rare in Denmark.

Tall, handsome, with a square jaw framed by wire-rimmed glasses and graying hair combed to the side, Poul Thorsen had shot out of

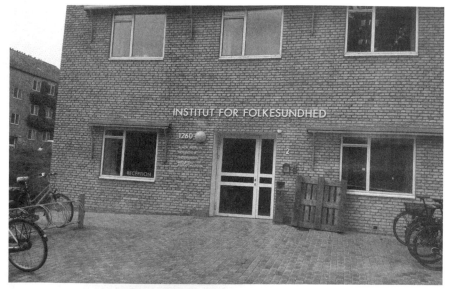

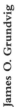

Aarhus University's Epidemiology Research Center, where Poul Thorsen used to work before he moved his research group NANEA off campus; and today where ex-CDC scientist Diana Schendel now works full time.

the shadow of research obscurity in his late thirties, just two years after earning his PhD. That trajectory won him the ire and jealousy of other doctors at AU—as Aarhus University is also known—who had far more expertise, experience, and a better network. Or so they believed. But Dr. Thorsen had one thing on his labcoat-wearing rivals. He had a vision that would match the trend at the start of the 21st century—mine vast pools of government health information for big data analytics—to the need of the U.S. Centers of Disease Control and Prevention (CDC). He would leverage troves of primary care data to fast-track studies.

Poul Thorsen was the one who saw the opportunity to exploit the Danish Health Registries—more than 200 national healthcare databases that store virtually all diseases, disorders, and ailments of Danish citizens born after 1968. It was what he had done during the 1990s in the Danish university hospital system and as a visiting research scientist at the CDC by the end of the decade in Atlanta, Georgia. He, with his colleagues, researched and backtested data for dozens of studies on everything from cerebral palsy and preterm delivery issues to autism and alcoholism.

Research studies, he knew, were faster, cheaper, and had less complications than running clinical trials, which were time- and labor-intensive in recruiting, interviewing, and babysitting patients. Poul Thorsen could fast-track studies that often took years at the clinical trial level, do it in a third of the time at a reduced cost, and produce better, if not more accurate, results. It "tied the economy of both healthcare authorities and providers to confer the final register with a high degree of completeness."[24]

A decade earlier, Thorsen knew "the register had so far only been used occasionally for research purposes. To take advantage of the register for research purposes within clinical and health services research, however, one must possess not only a detailed knowledge of Danish society, including the structure of the Danish healthcare system, but also an intimate acquaintance with rather complex agreement system and the actual interpretation of this."[25]

Poul Thorsen possessed both the domain and cultural knowledge. But better than his ability to conduct research, it was his Midas touch to raise grant funding from foundations, non-profit organizations, universities, and government agencies in Denmark and abroad that separated him from his older rivals and peers.

So Jørgen Jørgensen reread the statement one more time about a person he had never met. Just after April 1, 2009, his first day on the job at Aarhus University, the new director was plunged headlong in the investigation over forged CDC invoices billed to Thorsen's research

---

[24] Danish Medical Bulletin, 1997 Sept. 44(4):44953. "The Danish National Health Service Register. A tool for primary health care research." Olivarius NF et al.

[25] Ibid.

group. Other invoices had also been sent to Sahlgrenska University Hospital, part of the University of Gothenburg, Gothenburg, Sweden. When the dust settled, more than $1 million in CDC grant money went missing by the way of AU.

Where did it go? Jørgensen wondered.

Pensive, he sat back, removed his glasses, and rubbed his dry eyes as he recalled the words he said for his press release when he accepted the AU job a year earlier in February 2009: "Aarhus University is a very active and exciting workplace with a strong professional environment, and I look forward to being a part of it."[26]

He didn't realize how "active" or "exciting" it would be with the Thorsen probe blindsiding him. But with Thorsen canvassing consulting jobs, still claiming to be associated with AU, something had to be done to contain, if not reel in, the fallen doctor. Thorsen not only used other people's money, but other people's data, too.

Jørgen Jørgensen read the paragraph at top of the second page:

In March 2009, Dr. Thorsen resigned his faculty position at Aarhus University. In the meantime, it has come to the attention of Aarhus University that Dr. Thorsen has continued to act in such a manner as to create the impression that he still retains a connection to Aarhus University after the termination of his employment by the university. Furthermore, it has come to the attention of Aarhus University that Dr. Poul Thorsen has held full-time positions at both Emory University and Aarhus University simultaneously. Dr. Thorsen's double Full-time employment was unauthorized by Aarhus University, and he

---

[26] Dagens Medicin (Feb. 24, 2009) "Jørgen Jørgensen is the Director of the University of Aarhus," press release.

engaged in this employment situation despite the express prohibition of Aarhus University.[27]

The director picked up a pen and signed the highly unusual statement for a university. But then it was for a highly unusual, enigmatic, if successful, scientist.

---

[27] "Aarhus University Statement on Poul Thorsen," (Jan. 22, 2010) Jørgen Jørgensen.

# 3

# IN SCANDINAVIA LESS IS MORE

The 1973 oil crisis impacted the United States with long gas lines, forcing President Richard Nixon to sign the "Emergency Daylight Saving Time Energy Conservation Act," which would last two years. In Scandinavia, the energy crisis lit a fire under the fragility of national security for both Norway and Denmark. Overnight, energy independence became an Achilles' heel they could no longer ignore, not with World War II just a generation in the rearview mirror.

In Norway, they accelerated offshore oil and gas drilling plans from the 1960s by building state-of-the-art platforms and towing them out to sea. The aim was not only to become energy independent as a nation, but also to one day grow into an energy exporter. That day arrived early this century, while Norway also built up the largest sovereign wealth fund in the world, valued at $882 billion dollars of global assets.[28]

For Denmark, the tale was tactically different but grounded in the same long-term strategic goal of energy independence. With fewer offshore claims, the Danes decided to harness what they had in abundance—clean, green, sustainable wind. Denmark, not the Netherlands,

---

[28] http://www.swfinstitute.org/fund-rankings/

made the switch to Big Wind first and is today the world leader in that renewable energy category, according to Iver Høj Nielsen, the head of press at Denmark's www.stateofgreen.com. The State of Green is a public-private partnership (P3) tasked with "making Denmark fossil fuel independent by 2050," he said.

Since the oil crisis, Denmark has applied a "green" approach to business, living, transportation, and the health of its citizens. Beyond the Danish Health Registries cataloging citizens' ailments and diseases, the Danish government with the century-old Statens Serum Institut (SSI), the health agency responsible for both ensuring vaccine safety, as well as manufacturing vaccines and their components, heeded the advice of Hans Wigzell. Dr. Wigzell was the managing director at the National Swedish Bacteriological Laboratory in Stockholm, Sweden, from 1986–1991 and was a member of the Nobel Committee for Physiology or Medicine for a few years starting in 1987.

The Danish health authorities received Wigzell's brief, "Difficult to Substitute Mercury as a Preservative in Bacterial Vaccines," which he wrote in late 1990. By March 26, 1991, Maurice R. Hilleman, wrote a confidential seven-page cover letter to Dr. Gordon Douglas, then director of strategic planning for vaccine research at the National Institutes for Health (NIH). It highlighted Wigzell's findings. The subject of the letter: "Vaccine Task Force Assignment, Thimerosal (Merthiolate) Preservative Problems, Analysis, Suggestions for Resolution."

But the letter didn't come from any mere doctor or professor. Dr. Maurice R. Hilleman has been described as the "most successful vaccineologist in history."[29] In 1988, President Ronald Reagan presented Hilleman with the National Medal of Science. And Hilleman has been credited with saving more lives in the twentieth century than any medical

---

[29] Maugh, Thomas H., II (April 13, 2005), "Maurice R. Hilleman, 85; Scientist Developed Many Vaccines That Saved Millions of Lives" (http://articles.latimes.com/2005/apr/13/local/me-hilleman13), *Los Angeles Times*. Retrieved 2010-10-20.

scientist.[30] Maurice Hilleman invented eight out of the fourteen vaccines that populate the U.S. childhood immunology schedule today.

At the top of the confidential letter to Dr. Gordon Douglas, Hilleman didn't beat around the proverbial bush. There was no soft introduction or small talk. The first line read "1. Problem."

> The regulatory control agencies in some countries, particularly Scandinavia (especially Sweden), but also U.K. Japan, and Switzerland, have expressed concern for thimerosal, a mercurial preservative, in vaccines.
>
> Some countries require absence of thimerosal from single-dose vials and prefer to buy vaccines in the single-dose package. This trend will probably spread. Thimerosal is allowed where multidose vials are the only alternative.
>
> Sweden is requiring thimerosal-free single-dose packaging of all products, as soon as can be reasonably achieved. The deadline for DT is January, 1992.
>
> Competitor HibTITER (free of thimerosal) will be chosen for Haemophilus Influenzae vaccination until alternative thimerosal-free packaged vaccines are available.
>
> The U.S. Food & Drug Administration (CBER:Centers for Biological Evaluation and Research) does not have this concern for thimerosal but will permit exclusion from single-dose vials if requested and qualified. Misuse of single-dose vials by multiple puncture to achieve more does (e.g., 25 ug quantities for infants from 10 ug adult product) is the user's responsibility and ends with the requirement that the labeling clearly states that the vial contains a single dose and the vial is not to be reentered.
>
> The key issue is whether thimerosal, in the amount giver with the vaccine, does or does not constitute a safety hazard. However, perception of hazard may be equally important.

---

[30] Ibid

The confidential letter went on to discuss 2) "Composition of Thimerosal," 3) "Why the Concern? Thimerosal has been used for decades," 4) "Clinical Concerns" that focused on allergies and amalgam restorations found in dental work, 5) "Relative Toxicity of Mercurials," 6) "Toxicological Assessment of the Hazard of Thimerosal in the Amount Used," and 7) "Perspective and Conclusion."

Maurice Hilleman went on to recommend in 7b), "Combine as many vaccines as possible into a single-dose product so as to minimize the cumulative total mercury administered in multiple dosing." He suggested a potential solution for one vaccine, Pedvax HIB, to "consider the dried antigen as a single dose (which is thimerosal-free)."

Maurice R. Hilleman's final note read:

"Note, however, that Wigzell mentions only thimerosal-preserved DTP or DT given in at least 3 doses since the 1950s. Even with such small exposure, Sweden is moving as expeditiously as feasible to achieve a zero input of mercury from thimerosal. – M.R.H."

Denmark and Norway quickly followed Sweden's lead. By spring 1992, the last batches of vaccines containing thimerosal had been discontinued.

In Hans Wigzell's paper, Maurice Hilleman, Dr. Gordon Douglas and thirteen other U.S. health officials, scientists, and doctors ignored his recommendations outlined in the brief on thimerosal:

- "There are however no investigations that show that there is a difference in general toxicity when the uptake of mercury is from the stomach-intestines or after injections."
- "There are also reports of general reactions in patients treated with mercury-containing medications. This should be studied in relation to the tremendous large number of subjects vaccinated with preparations containing thimerosal sodium."
- "Our goal is to develop, as soon as possible, vaccines completely free of mercury."

Unfortunately, Maurice Hilleman didn't emphasize conducting either study, nor did he recommend to Dr. Douglas or the NIH that the

United States should follow the Scandinavian countries in making vaccines thimerosal-free by 1992.

Why did Maurice Hilleman, a world leading vaccineologist, have not even the slightest trace of human curiosity to find out why the Swedish bacteriologist took such a firm stand against thimerosal? Why didn't he want to find out why Wigzell persuaded Japan and the other Scandinavian countries to remove the mercury preservative from all vaccines that contained the toxic substance?

"Hilleman's biggest concern was for Merck to quickly qualify to produce the Hg-free single DT doses for Scandinavia—and not lose that market and its money," wrote F. Edward Yazbak, MD, in an email. Dr. Yazbak had practiced pediatrics and was a school physician in northern Rhode Island for more three decades. He also has an autistic grandson.

So had the "greatest vaccineologist" and the doctor who "saved more lives in the twentieth century than any other medical scientist" worded his cover letter differently, then the collision course that the vaccine–autism divide would create a decade later would never have happened. Unfortunately, as scientist working for a pharmaceutical giant, his first job was to making money for his firm. He never questioned why mercury in vaccines had suddenly become a concern after a half century of apparently "safe use"—maybe it was due to the sharp increase in the number of vaccines, thus creating an accumulative or a "snowball" effect. He ended up putting Dr. Poul Thorsen, his future CDC girlfriend Diana Schendel, and the CDC executives on a collision course, where "playing ball" and "collusion" would become the operative words. They were the same executives charged with protecting the health of American children; all they would end up doing was try to exonerate mercury as a preservative in vaccines and label it "safe," as if it was a can of tuna fish.

Then maybe the nearly $2 million in grants and missing funds that Poul Thorsen would one day be indicted for stealing wouldn't have happened either.

But that's a story for a parallel universe.

# 4

# DOCTORS OF THE HUMAN ENVIRONMENT

Poul Bak Thorsen was born on Monday, May 1, 1961.

"May Day," which held no special holiday in Denmark that year, had a different ring and feel to it across the Atlantic Ocean. On the same day as Thorsen's mother gave birth, the new communist government of Cuba celebrated its victory and rise to power with a fourteen-hour parade after having survived President John F. Kennedy's botched Bay of Pigs military operation, which had failed two weeks earlier to overthrow Fidel Castro's regime.

Poul Thorsen never quite fit the socialist model, despite being born and raised in Denmark, a socialist culture and government. Yet he wasn't any ordinary medical student. He had no interest in being one of Denmark's 1,500 general practitioners a quarter of a century ago. Nor did he ever commit to any particular field of study, any one medical specialty, such as oncology, or make any long-term plan in terms of a medical career. He was neither fickle nor feckless, as much as he possessed a lust to feed a voracious appetite for research and knowledge. Instead, he would dabble his talents and sharp analytical mind across an array of subjects, diseases, and disorders, whether in the mind (autism), the nervous system (cerebral palsy), or the womb (preterm delivery issues). Not wanting to be boxed in, Poul Thorsen was more Apple's Steve Jobs, who was a born leader and generalist, than Vincent van Gogh, who was an experimenter that would later in his short life become a specialist—but without the talents of either the tech designer or Impressionist painter.

Since his first project at Aarhus University Hospital, Department of Clinical Medicine in 1987 as a medical doctoral student, Poul Thorsen would graduate with a masters of science in medicine in 1989 and begin training as an intern to earn his "MD" title, according to an email that confirmed part of Thorsen's education by Thayan Rajagopaian, an administrative officer at Uddannelse Educational Law at Aarhus University.

During his three years as a medical doctor intern at Denmark's largest health science institute, which covered many medical specialties across a network of research centers and a vast university hospital system, Poul Thorsen would become the principal investigator (PI) on his first study about a rare form of female cancer. (Ovarian tumors caused by metastatic tumors of the appendix; two case reports, by Poul Thorsen, Helle Dybdahl, Helmer Søgård, and Birger R. Møller, MD, University Hospital, Sygehuset.) The study, which was submitted to the *European Journal of Obstetrics & Gynecology and Reproductive Biology*, was accepted for publication on June 6, 1990.

The little five-page study on just two middle-aged patients, with a thin ten medical references, would appear a year later in the *European Journal of Medical Sciences.*

The paper opened:

Malignant tumors of the appendix are seldom reported. Most common among these rare tumors are the carcinoid, which must be distinguished from the extremely rare true adenocarcinoma. These tumors present in most cases with symptoms similar to acute appendicitis, but may also appear with clinical manifestations similar to rupture of an inflamed appendix, intra-abdominal tumor or right-sided lower quadrant masses.

The paper concluded in the "Discussion" section:

Previously only 30 cases of primary adenocarcinomas or adenocarcinomas in the vermiform appendix metastasizing to the
ovary have been described [5-9]. The metastatic spread from
the appendix to the ovary in the two cases presented is possibly by the peritoneal route involving a localized peritonitis
carcinomatosa.]

Why did Poul Thorsen choose such a rare—only thirty previous primary cases—form of cancer that took root in the appendix
of women and spread to the ovaries? The appendix, as science once
believed incorrectly, appeared to be an evolutionary dead end. But a
recent Duke University study said: "The lowly appendix, long-regarded
as a useless evolutionary artifact, won newfound respect two years ago
(2007) when researchers proposed that it actually serves a critical function. The appendix, they said, is a safe haven where good bacteria could
hang out until they were needed to repopulate the gut after a nasty case
of diarrhea, for example."[31]

Why was cancer of the female appendix important to Poul
Thorsen? Was it to work closely with his two mentors, Drs. Søgård
and Møller? Would that experience lead to other areas of research on
the human anatomy?

Over the next quarter century, Poul Thorsen led as principal
investigator or co-authored more than 100 research studies, many of
them using data mined from the Danish Health Registries. In these
published studies, Thorsen would never do another study on appendix cancer, nor would he develop his medical specialty in oncology.
Helmer Søgård would go on with a distinguished medical career
at Aarhus University until his death in June 2013, while Dr. Birger
Møller would continue to be involved with Poul Thorsen's medical

---

[31] Science Daily, August 21, 2009, Duke University Medical Center.

research over the next fifteen years, in which they worked on several key studies together.

By 1992, after earning his MD, Dr. Poul Thorsen headed for the big city of Copenhagen and joined world-renowned Statens Serum Institut, the national R&D institution and vaccine manufacturer. There he would spend the next three years of his career researching and datamining the Danish National Birth Cohort—aka the Danish Health Registries. At SSI, Thorsen expanded his taste for the medically unusual and the anomaly as if to challenge his mind, placate his intellect, and push the boundaries of his knowledge on such diverse subjects as venereal disease, alcoholism, and cellular level forms of cancer and other diseases.

What was the connection between dissimilar diseases?

The data of his fellow countrymen—their physical and mental deficits, their diseases and disorders, their odd ailments and genetic flaws—became his lens, his encyclopedia on all that was not well in Denmark. The little-used collective of over 200 regional and national databases from the homogenized society of more than five million people would be used to reflect the flaws of and threats to much larger populations found in other nations, such as the United States. One day he would capitalize on all of that "free" Danish data he had access to as a medical scientist.

With the entire country as his cohort—defined as "a group of patients examined or treated together"—Thorsen, like a young Alexander the Great, knew his domain, his Denmark. His capitalist tastes in a socialist-leaning country weren't big enough to contain his appetite or ambition to become rich or slake his thirst for knowledge, medical—abnormal, and all points in between.

★   ★   ★

Born in 1955, Diana Elizabeth Schendel was the oldest of four children born and raised in Tallahassee, Florida. Her parents—Margaret Ruth

Wise, a nurse, and Larry Schendel—were hardworking Americans from Louisiana. The children had the privilege of growing up in Los Robles Gate, a historic section of Tallahassee. The family house was "nominated for the National Registry of Historic Places, was the site of civil rights movie-filming, weddings, and wedding receptions for many family and friends and hosting of visiting dignitaries to Florida State University such a former Secretary of State Dean Rusk and the First Lady of American Theater, Helen Hayes," according to her mother's obituary.[32]

Growing up at the intersection of Floridian history and a major U.S. college town—today with some 70,000 students who attend Florida A&M University and Florida State University combined—branded an indelible mark in Diana Schendel's young mind. After graduating Leon High School in Tallahassee in 1972, she never left America's 128th largest city. Instead, she attended Florida State University (FSU). It would take her six interrupted years to complete her double major with bachelor of science degrees in biology and anthropology, her first love, even though she would graduate magna cum laude and be elected to the Phi Beta Kappa sorority.

In Article III, "Election to Membership," the 2009 Phi Beta Kappa bylaws require:

(d) Members in course shall be elected as described below from among Florida

State University juniors and seniors who meet the following criteria:

(i) Whether elected as juniors or seniors, potential members must:

1) Exhibit scholarly achievement, good character, and varied intellectual *and cultural interests*.

---

[32] *The Times and Democrat*, "Obituary of Diana Ruth Wise Schendel, Atlanta," GA, May 8, 2008.

The high threshold for membership—grade, character, intellect—into Phi Beta Kappa was in existence during the 1970s just as
it is today. According to Schendel's CDC employment application
affidavit she swore and signed, her undergraduate studies included
biology/health sciences and anthropology. Why did it take Diana
Schendel, a local from a wealthy enclave of Tallahassee who was
bright and possessed good character, six years to complete her
undergraduate study?

From 1972 until she graduated from FSU in 1977, Diana Elizabeth
Schendel married not once, but twice. Both to older men. Both of whom
were research scientists at FSU. They might as well have been from the
neighborhood she grew up in with her siblings in Los Robles Gate.

Her first marriage was to Donald Lewis Crusoe, a lifelong anthropologist born in 1943 who published his first paper on the "Study
of Aboriginal Trade: a Petrographic Analysis of Certain Ceramic
Types from Florida" in 1969 at FSU. But he was married once
before to Sarah Crusoe; they divorced on Wednesday, November 22,
1972—the day before Thanksgiving, and the same year he earned
his PhD at the University of Georgia with a thesis on "Interaction
Networks and New World Fiber Tempered Pottery." Two years and
one month later to the day, Crusoe married Diana Schendel on
Sunday, December 22, 1974, in a Tallahassee wedding. As an anthropologist researcher he was either naive of American holidays, when
stresses run high in families, or needed to cleanse his life of his ex-
wife by getting married during winter break before the next semester started in the new year.

Of medium height and slender build, with light brown hair and
a smile that flashed a Michael Strahan gap in her front teeth, Diana
Schendel Crusoe left her sorority Phi Beta Kappa not to merely settle
down and begin a family with her new husband or attend school to
earn her degree but to learn from a mentor in anthropology. As much
as they had a passion for the same discipline, feeding off one another
with each new path of research and discovery, it went against type

for a couple with different tastes and personalities, or as the saying goes "opposites attract." With the combination of being married to a much older man as a college coed and sharing little more than pre-twentieth century human artifacts in Florida, Diana Schendel moved on from Donald Crusoe to finish her studies, and then got divorced.

Finding another older man on Florida State campus with a similar interest in scientific research in archaeologist, Christopher Everett Hamilton, born in 1947 in Suwanee, GA, brought Schendel's undergraduate studies to a close. Earning her double major in 1977, she went on to marry husband number two on Saturday, November 5, 1977.

But for the same reasons her first marriage to Donald Crusoe failed, her second marriage in less than a decade to Hamilton would dissolve quickly, too. Either unaware or bearing a blindspot from being the oldest sibling in the rough-and-tumble decade of the 1970s Diane was, to a degree, socially inept, unable to date a boyfriend for a few years first, maybe even live with him to see if their partnership would work and flourish, and instead getting hitched twice to one research scientist after another. Those relationships limited her understanding of how the private world, with all its ambition and competitive juices, really worked.

By the end of the decade, it was clear Schendel needed a change in scenery. She needed time and space from dating men that were her mirror image; she knew deep down that marriage and raising a family of her own might not be in the cards for her.

Diana moved to State College, Pennsylvania, or "Happy Valley" as it is known on the Penn State University campus and some 87 miles west of the state capital, Harrisburg. The twice-divorced research student attended another major college football school, home to late Coach Joe Paterno's Nittany Lions and the same college program in which defensive coordinator Jerry Sandusky sodomized boys when he wasn't scheming defenses for the next game, which was once in a while against FSU.

In 1980, Diana Schendel earned a masters of the arts in anthropology. Her dissertation focused on "Age Changes in Blood Pressure

Among Three Populations of Samoan Children." It would make it
into a fiftieth anniversary of the American Association of Physical
Anthropologists (AAPA), in the "Proceedings of the Fiftieth Annual
Meeting of AAPA" held in Detroit, Michigan, April 22–25, 1981,
published by John Wiley & Sons.

With Samoans becoming her focus during the 1980s at Penn State,
she shed her twice-divorced past, moving her anthropological research
far from the humans and cultures that populated pre-white man Florida
to the cultures and people of the South Pacific islands. By 1989, she
finished her doctoral thesis on sex differences in factors associated with
body fatness in Western Samoans, and earned her PhD from Penn State
University.

A decade on, researching the Samoan people in State College,
Diana Schendel scrubbed both of her married names from her life
and looked to move once more—this time taking a research position at Tufts University in the autumn of 1990. Before she made the
move, Diana and fifteen other PhD candidates with dissertations on
the Pacific traveled to Hawaii for the nineteenth annual meeting of
the Association for Social Anthropology in Oceania. Given a tight
window of a week during spring break, the postdoctoral grads traveled from the Aloha State to islands important to their specific areas of
research.[33]

Leaving Penn State for Tufts University in Boston, Massachusetts,
Schendel began her career as an assistant professor in the department
of sociology and anthropology, but that job, which didn't pay well,
wouldn't last long.

On November 14, 1990, the state of Massachusetts hired Diana
Schendel to become a senior epidemiologist for the Woburn
Environment and Birth Study (WEBS). A clear departure from

---

[33] 1989-90 AAA *Guide to Departments of Anthropology, Penn State University.*

everything she had done in the past in terms of research, wedlock, and education since stepping onto Florida State campus in the fall of 1972, the PhD in anthropology moved far away from the cultures of people to the human environment and how the body, toxins, and carcinogens impact the lives of pregnant women and their offspring they raise into children.

The location of the new epidemiological research was a U.S. Superfund site.

Woburn, Massachusetts, a small town located nine miles north of Boston with a population one-sixth the size of Tallahassee, sat at the center of the Industrial Revolution more than a century ago. First, it was home to tanneries and all their pollutants and run-off from chemical processes; then after World War II, big business plants of Beatrice Foods and W.R. Grace & Company, a "high-performance specialty chemical and materials" manufacturer for the construction industry, opened shop. Those two companies were at the center of a civil lawsuit brought on by the parents of children caught in a mysterious leukemia cluster on the east side of town where two new wells, G and H, built in the mid-1960s, were found to be polluted with toxins and carcinogens. Author and professor Jonathan Harr captured all of that and much more in his bestselling book *A Civil Action*, which in 1996 was turned into a Hollywood movie starring John Travolta as the attorney for the plaintiffs.

What caused the cancer cluster? Was it unknown toxins? And what was in the drinking water of wells G and H? To find out, the CDC joined WEBS to produce back-tested, researched childhood epidemiological studies in the east part of Woburn on those children who were stricken by leukemia and those who were not.

Hired away from Tufts as senior epidemiologist, Diana Schendel began work on the biostatistics of the cancer cluster, assessing human health effects on children from the wells that were polluted. WEBS work was separate from the civil lawsuit.

"The WEBS is an epidemiologic study designed to assess the effects of potential exposure to toxic environmental substances on the reproductive health of the Boston suburban community. It consists of three primary study components:

1) "A 20-year retrospective study to assess the prevalence of adverse reproductive outcomes, including congenital malformations, in Woburn relative to a number of referent populations;

2. "A prospective surveillance study to assess the current prevalence of these outcomes relative to the referent populations, and;

3) "A retrospective study to assess the prevalence of adverse reproductive outcomes in Woburn relative to the level of exposure of residents to the contaminated municipal water supply."

She split her time on the study between "conducting all of the epidemiologic analysis and collaboration on all scientific components of the study, to the supervision of reproductive health outcome data collection, data management, and computer programming staff, and report preparation and presentation to both public and professional audiences."[34]

After two years of working at WEBS, in which her starting salary of $40,000 climbed to $48,000 per annum,[35] the CDC lured Diana Schendel away from the Woburn study, which wouldn't publish its first report until 1994 and a final report in 1996. For Schendel, working at the CDC enabled her to pursue her postdoctoral career in epidemiology, even though she never studied it beyond a couple

---

[34] Diana Schendel, CDC Application Affidavit for Employment, November 1992.

[35] Diana Schendel, CDC Appointment Affidavits, April 19, 1993.

of undergraduate courses at FSU in the 1970s. More importantly, Schendel could move back south to her roots where she would work in Atlanta, Georgia, just north of where she grew up and went to school in the panhandle of Florida.

The odd thing about her stint at WEBS is one can no longer find a record of her working in Woburn in any of her resumes post-2004. That includes both her resumes at the CDC and a variety of sub-agency or non-profit organizations she worked for, as well as her new career as a senior research epidemiologist on autism studies at Aarhus University—Poul Thorsen's old undergraduate medical stomping ground and where he would one day gain notoriety by the turn of the millennium by launching a university research group within the university with CDC money.

# 5

# AGENT ORANGE IS THE NEW BLACK

In fall of 1998, the CDC accepted Poul Thorsen as a postdoctoral visiting scientist to its Atlanta headquarters in its soon-to-be-formed National Center of Birth Defects and Developmental Disabilities (NCBDDD). Dr. Thorsen researched and wrote his PhD thesis, "Bacterial Vaginosis in Pregnancy: A Population-based Study," at the University of Southern Denmark (SDU) in Odense, Denmark. It's the Scandinavian country's third largest city on the island of Funen, about one hundred miles southwest of Copenhagen, and an hour and a half south by train from Denmark's second largest city Aarhus, which translates to "Year-House."

His thesis struck a chord with the CDC since Thorsen used the technique of mining the Danish Health Registries to support research findings and draw conclusions. The backtesting of data was something Dr. Diana Schendel did eight years earlier in conjunction with the CDC on the leukemia cluster at the Woburn Superfund Site. But Dr. Schendel did her epidemiological analysis from a hodgepodge of analog files; hospital, school, and residential recordkeeping; meetings with parents and residents; follow up interviews; and other static, fragmented data from an assortment of historical and archival records.

What Poul Thorsen had done was wholly different. He conducted deep dives into digital information, which was stored in several national and regional databases. That streamlined his research and fast-tracked studies, avoiding the labor-intensive logistics-drag and steep costs of performing actual clinical trials using real patients. General practitioners and patients alike—with no financial motivation one way or another to cheat the system, as Denmark claims—entered the data and that supposedly reduced human input errors for Denmark's unique national cohort.

But like any manmade system with multiple entry points, timely data inputs, and human error—fatigue, distraction, bias such as being bitter at the healthcare system, or dishonesty—the Danish Health Registries was neither perfect nor infallible nor 100 percent accurate.

The other impressive half of Poul Thorsen's research background was his scientific studies on venereal disease of Greenlanders, Greenland being a Danish colony—oral contraceptives, post-abortion and stillbirth with mothers suffering from infections; sterility in the uterine cavity, microorganisms of bacterial vaginosis, and cervical cancer. But the CDC's human resources recruiter must have overlooked reading the fine print of Dr. Thorsen's published studies. Had the person done that, the recruiter might have noticed an issue that arose in a study and subsequent rebuttal published in *Lancet* (Feb. 1997) on "Sensitivity of Ligase Chain Reaction Assay of Urine from Pregnant Women for Chlamydiatrachomatis," with coauthors Inge anum and one of Thorsen's mentors, Dr. Birger R. Møller.

The authors' reply:

SIR—We are surprised by Muldoon's comments. Ours was a collaborative study with Abbott Laboratories and they were offered coauthorship of the paper but never replied. We found that the LCR assay applied to urine samples from pregnant women did not work as well as an enzyme immunoassay on cervical swabs. The result was clear-cut and we saw no scientific reason for expanding the scope of the project by, for example, comparing findings in non-pregnant women. When this study began there were no transport instructions for urine samples; the 18–24 h uncooled transport used was well known to the project collaborators.[36]

(Muldoon was the letter writer to the *Lancet* editor that spurred Dr. Thorsen to write a response.)

Nearly twenty years after the study was conducted, Abbott Laboratories, which is headquartered in Illinois and has an office in Denmark, didn't respond to emails and calls to verify whether they ever did the lab work claimed by Poul Thorsen and the other two authors for the study. Although Poul Thorsen had impressive credentials for a postdoctoral visiting scientist, with respect to the CDC's Birth Defects division he still had not worked in two specific areas of infant maladies that would come to define his career: cerebral palsy and autism.

When Poul Thorsen heard the husky voice, deeper than normal for the slender, diminutive, well-dressed Diana Schendel, for the first time, he was aroused and curious. He noted there was no wedding band or diamond ring on the ring finger of her left hand. His much larger 6' 2" frame straightened in her presence; his spine stiffened. He felt blood flow, warming his face flush, making him light headed. His mind raced as he gazed into her light blue eyes, graced by an inviting smile and her dusty brown, shoulder-length hair. In a word, the twice-divorced epidemiologist disarmed Thorsen. In the Southern belle he saw not only an opportunity to get laid when he was over in the United States, but he also believed she could be his Otis Elevator ride in advancing his career without the usual wait of a young doctor

---

[36] *Lancet*, Vol. 349, April 5, 1997 (pg. 1,025).

or the friction of bowing to senior university professors on both sides of the Atlantic.

But it was Diana Schendel's voice, an octave lower, a bit gravelly that, when matched with her charming face and smallish size body, wooed Thorsen with thoughts of pleasure and possible courtship.

He would quickly learn about her PhD work in anthropology, her epidemiology studies in Woburn on the leukemia cluster, and her being lured away from the WEBS cancer cluster study to join the CDC in 1992. Poul Thorsen also learned that the woman he was attracted to was six years his senior. And yet he, the junior in their budding relationship, had published several more studies than she had at that point of their careers. What he didn't know at the time of meeting the scientist, however, was that he would co-author more than three dozen studies over the next fifteen years. Over that span, Diana Schendel's job title would change a couple of times, and with suspected demotions, there was an apparent cut in base pay. Why was she demoted? What was in her past research or in being a team player that the CDC felt compelled to mold her into the likeness of her boss Dr. Coleen Boyle, who was a master manipulator in her own right. At the dawn of the Internet and World Wide Web in the mid-1990s, Dr. Boyle's past work with Agent Orange epidemiological studies for the CDC was more or less hidden from Schendel and other peers outside of her division.

From 1998 through 1999, Dr. Diana Schendel would serve as a supervisory epidemiologist under Dr. Coleen Boyle.

When Thorsen met Boyle for the first time, he saw a focused, serious, but banal-looking scientist in the body of a librarian. With short brown hair, thick eyebrows, and an expressionless face, Dr. Boyle was all business, no charm—a true bureaucrat. She and Schendel had worked together with other CDC scientists on a pair of studies on the "Prevalence of Selected Developmental Disabilities in Children 3-10 Years of Age" (1996), and the "Risk of Cerebral Palsy or Mental Retardation Among Very Low-Birth-Weight Children Aged 3 to 5 Years" (1997). Later that year, Diana Schendel, as principal investigator, would follow up that study with the relation study between "Very Low-Birth-Weight and Development Delay among Preschool Children without Disabilities."

As Poul Thorsen shared stories, techniques, and his studies on diseases about mothers with Diana Schendel, he saw the other side to the ailing mother equation—babies suffering from birth defects, diseases, and disorders such as autism. Their backgrounds complemented each other's. In Poul Thorsen, Diana saw a new masculine man a scientist, who was younger than either one of her staid PhD husbands from the 1970s. The Dane was a breath of fresh air, a candle flame that she could cultivate in her life where together they could help each other get ahead and solve some of the greater challenges impacting the health and development of babies, infants, and children worldwide. It was a noble endeavor.

For Poul Thorsen, ever the opportunist with an envious eye on big, rich United States, the land of opportunity, home to the American dream and capitalism, securing the visiting scientist slot at the CDC that year was more than a boon; he got lucky with Diana Schendel, too. Poul landed in the right department—the up-and-coming Division of Birth Defects and Developmental Disabilities—while meeting an available—no, a needy—American scientist he could bed for pleasure and corporate gain. Add Diana Schendel's boss, Coleen Boyle, to the serendipitous overseas assignment, and Poul grasped that he could learn how to operate inside the renowned U.S. agency in charge of the healthcare of more than 275 million people.

Dr. Boyle received her master of science sygiene in biostatistics and her PhD in epidemiology from the University of Pittsburgh's School of Public Health. She followed up her health sciences education with postdoctoral training in epidemiological studies at Yale University. But after her first year at the CDC in 1984, the "Librarian" would spend the rest of the decade working on the congressional Agent Orange prevalence reporting team. Coleen Boyle served as the principal investigator for the Agent Orange studies on Vietnam veterans.

The dioxin-loaded Agent Orange defoliant earned its name for the orange stripe wrapped around the fifty-five-gallon drum of the toxic chemical. During Operation Ranch Hand in the Vietnam War, the U.S. Air Force rarely diluted the chemical, thereby increasing its short-term (cancer) and long-term (DNA) impacts on the health of the Vietnamese and U.S. troops in the jungles. But the Agent Orange studies, under the guidance and leadership of CDC, unlike the dioxin chemical, would be diluted, manipulating the veterans' health statistics with the aim to show "no association" as a trigger.

Like Diana Schendel's work at Woburn, based on the Monsanto patents, Dow Chemical manufactured Agent Orange at a half dozen plants across America; most of them would later become Superfund sites in the 1980s. The dioxin manufacturing plants included Dow Chemical, Midland, Michigan; Monsanto, Nitro, West Virginia; Diamond Alkali/Shamrock, Newark, New Jersey; Hercules, Jacksonville, Arkansas; Thompson-Hayward Chemical, Kansas City, Kansas; the U.S. Rubber Company/Uniroyal, Elmira, Ontario; Thompson Chemical Corp, St. Louis, Missouri; and Hoffman-Tuff, Inc., Verona, Missouri.[37]

"At the time CDC was diluting the study, using the rationale that the Defense Department's records were inaccurate or missing, a team of expert scientists from the National Academy or Sciences' Institute of Medicine (IOM) made a site visit to the Department's Environmental Support Group (ESG). The scientific data, found the ESG records important and useable, and was critical of CDC's performance."—In other words, for omitting data, as the CDC stated it could not fill the "gaps" in the Department records, when in fact the scientific team said it could do just that.[38]

---

[37] "The Agent Orange Record Map," www.agentorangerecord.com/information/what_is_dioxin/sites/

[38] "The Agent Orange Coverup: A Case of Flawed Science and Political Manipulation, the Twelfth Report by the Committee on Government Operations," together with Dissenting Views, Pg. 19 (Aug. 9, 1990) 101st Congress.

Beyond shutting down the Agent Orange study in 1987, halfway into the project, the Reagan White House didn't want the U.S. to be liable for the tens of thousands of injured troops exposed to dioxin. Thus, the CDC team, led by Dr. Coleen Boyle, found ways to bury, skew, and scatter the data to show no correlation between the aerosol flights by the U.S. Air Force and the U.S. troops on the ground. Dr. Boyle served "as the principal investigator for the Vietnam Experience mortality studies and as senior epidemiologist for a large, multi-centered cancer case-control study."[39]

This is remarkable coming from a scientist, who would go on to earn the CDC Charles C. Shepard Award twice for scientific excellence in 1997 and 2004, on her way to being named director of the CDC's Birth Defects and Developmental Disorders unit when she found "nothing that showed a correlation between Agent Orange and the Vietnam veterans stricken with cancer. If she couldn't find a link between dioxin and cancer with Agent Orange, then how was Coleen Boyle ever going to find any toxic or environmental cause behind the autism epidemic a decade later?" a physician, with expertise on the pathology of diseases, asked out loud.

"Unfortunately, as hearings before the Human Resources and Intergovernmental Relations Subcommittee on July 11, 1989 revealed, the design, implementation, and conclusions of the CDC study were so ill conceived as to suggest that political pressures once again interfered with the kind of professional, unbiased review Congress had sought to obtain."[40]

Christian's testimony raised questions about the ability of the CDC staff to sufficiently comprehend and use the military record. He testified about being astounded when he discovered that CDC was identifying enemy locations when it thought it had pinpointed U.S. sites.

---

[39] From Dr. Coleen Boyle's Biography: http://www.cdc.gov/ncbddd/aboutus/biographies/boyle.html

[40] Admiral Elmo R. Zumwalt, May 5, 1990, declassified testimony before 101st Congress.

(Richard Christian was, the former director of the U.S. Army and Joint Services Environmental Surpport Group, Department of the Army.)

"At one point, the Centers for Disease Control attempted to take over the work of ESG (DoD Environmental Support Group) from the study. My staff provided the CDC with copies of daily journals. In a test, of that exercise, the personnel in the Centers for Disease Control recorded the grid points from the Viet Cong locations. Certainly we were not interested in the enemy locations; we were look for the U.S. locations and the U.S. grid points."[41]

In other words, by omitting data, CDC explained it could not fill in the gaps of the fragmented Department of Defense (DoD) records, when, on the contrary, the scientific team said it could do just that. But the CDC changed the criteria, search grids, and locations in the study the way a breeze turns a farmer's weathervane. Dr. Boyle must have thought they could fool the DoD topographers and Congress as well, since they wrongly believed they couldn't "accurately" line up the field sites in Vietnam when the Ranch Hand flights dispersed Agent Orange across the green jungle canopy.

It reminds one of when environmentalists accused BP, in response to its runaway oil spill in 2010, for sending night-time oil dispersant flights over the Gulf of Mexico to sink rather than "disperse" the oil. Today, the sunken oil carpets the bottom of the gulf in a two-inch thick black sludge that radiates in a twenty-five-mile ring from the Macondo Well, killing marine life on the seafloor. BP ended up paying $18.7 billion, according to a *Wall Street Journal* cover story on July 2, 2015.

Like BP, which deliberately under-estimated the oil spill rate in order to lower the government penalty, "using its criticism of the

---

[41] *The Agent Orange Coverup: A Case of Flawed Science and Political Manipulation, the Twelfth Report* by the Committee on Government Operations together with Dissenting Views, Pg. 13 (Aug. 9,1990) 101st Congress, 2nd Session.

ESG records as its excuse, the CDC and the AOWG (Agent Orange Working Group) were inclined against proceeding with the study."[42]

The "Agent Orange Coverup" report went on to call out that the breach of the study's protocol by the CDC by circumventing AWOG in the review process; that the CDC couldn't confirm whether the synthetic chemical dioxin had a "half-life" or not, and if so, how long it was; that it could not reach any conclusions on exposure because it could not develop a method to assess exposure; and that in the end, "any possible link between herbicide and the reported birth defects was dismissed by CDC because of the cancellation of the exposure study."[43]

This set the path forward to allow backroom deals between CDC and the White House to act like BP and sink the truth, showing no causation between the obvious Occam's razor connection between Agent Orange spraying in the jungles and the sharp rise in rare and acute cancers of Vietnam veterans.

"So strident was the administration in its belief that the Federal Government should not be liable for exposure to toxic chemicals that the Justice Department ordered the Defense Department to assist the Special Master overseeing the legal settlement between the manufacturers of Agent Orange and Vietnam veterans."[44]

The Agent Orange storm of political corruption set the stage for Dr. Coleen Boyle and others at the CDC on how to deal with the tsunami of autism cases that would explode across the U.S. by 1995 and continue to rise. Boyle learned, and likely taught Diana Schendel, how to move a political football around on sensitive public issues, leveraging the news media, steering public perception, working with or dominating other agencies, milking lobbyists, and above all, stonewalling Congress.

---

[42] Ibid 21.

[43] Ibid, pg. 33.

[44] Ibid, pg. 29.

So in the end, what were the taxpayer costs that the CDC burned through to produce "no findings" in the curtailed five-year Agent Orange study? According to the U.S. Accounting Office Briefing Report, it noted how the "CDC spent $51.5 of the $70.4 million it received from the Department of Veterans Affairs."[45]

Yet it canceled the Agent Orange study in 1987.

"CDC awarded two major contracts, worth $6.6 million, nearly 10% of total study budget for downtime, since its protocol and methodology on how to accurately identify Agent Orange wasn't developed yet, and that poor negotiating practices cost U.S taxpayers an additional $86,779 in increased contract costs. When inquiring why CDC canceled the Agent Orange Report, CDC stated that military records could not be used to accurately determine the exposure."[46]

"CDC used $33.2 million for contracts and interagency agreements to do the four studies."[47]

For producing nothing of significance, the CDC had its template of obfuscation. Unlike the U.S. Air Force, which kept impeccable records, the CDC knew that "20 million gallons of herbicides (11 million gallons of which was Agent Orange, most of which was undiluted) was sprayed from 1962–1970.[48]

For all of CDC's incompetence and deliberate masking of the truth, it would take another six years for the IOM to produce a 1996 report that finally somewhat linked Agent Orange to the risk of birth defects in Vietnamese veterans' children.[49] Of the six congressmen that signed the Dissenting View Report, Richard K. Armey's name at the

---

[45] "Agent Orange Studies: Poor Contracting Practices at Centers for Disease Control Increased Costs," (Sep. 28, 1990)

[46] Ibid, pg. 2.

[47] Ibid, pg. 15.

[48] Ibid, pg. 1.

[49] *JAMA* April 10, 1996—Vol. 175, No. 14, Joan Stephenson, PhD.

top would one day become the most controversial name in the autism community.

For Poul Thorsen, the politically machined Coleen Boyle gave him a template he would use later at CDC and the universities he worked with in Denmark. Seeing cracks in CDC's veneer and feeling its sense of desperation in getting ahead of the autism-vaccine crisis, Thorsen would exploit the weakness with the agency's executive management; Diana Schendel would be his meal ticket to the promised land he craved.

# 6

# THE BOYLE-ING POINT OF DATA

In the summer of 1999, the bad news for the CDC emerged quietly, percolating up from a shallow well of research in an abstract for a study that wouldn't be published for another four years after undergoing several permutations. The results, if made public, would be too damaging to the CDC's plan to expand and commoditize the U.S. immunization program. In Silicon Valley parlance, scale-and value-added benefits would be denied, not for the end user, but for the industry, the system, the monolith of money, and power.

The lead investigator, Dr. Thomas M. Verstraeten from Belgium, together with CDC coauthors D. Gu, Bob L. Davis, and Frank DeStefano (the project director for the Vaccine Safety Datalink and medical epidemiologist in the National Immunization Program (NIP), where he would one day be appointed acting chief of the Immunization Safety Branch of NIP in 2004) became the uneasy foreign scientist guns for hire.

The abstract was titled "Increased risk of developmental neurological impairment after high exposure to thimerosal-containing vaccine in first month of life."

Verstraeten, who ran the statistical analysis on thimerosal containing vaccines (TCV) for the study, wrote in a December email, titled "It Just Won't Go Away," "I added another exposure variable (addcat) in one list that looks at the increase of mercury each month for the first three months, divided by the average bodyweight in the first, second, and third month and takes the maximum value of this. This does not show much, to which I would conclude that, except for epilepsy, all of the harm is done in the first month."[50]

There it was: a sharp increase with TCV caused speech delays, body tics, fine motor impairments, and increased the likelihood for some babies to get brain damage.

If politics hadn't tainted the minds and leadership at the CDC, publishing that abstract in a full-blown study would have been the next logical step. But that didn't happen. The higher-ups in the CDC didn't like the results; they didn't want the link that clearly showed that ethylmercury of thimerosal, which is 49.6% mercury, caused neurodevelopmental issues in babies and infants. Earlier that summer, vaccine manufacturers in Merck and SmithKline Beecham had written letters voluntarily stating they would remove thimerosal from their vaccines that contained them, but the CDC ignored the offer, informing them that all systems were go with the manufacturing process.

By the next spring, Agent Orange expert Dr. Coleen Boyle got wind of the thimerosal controversy as the rates of autism in the United States skyrocketed from 1-in-10,000 to 1-in-150 babies born. Knowing the lessons from her infamous Agent Orange study that the CDC "couldn't accurately assess the field data," there would be no repercussion from Congress, no political fallout, zero penalties, and absolutely no firings. So Boyle took charge of steering the Verstraeten study months before the secret June Simpsonwood meeting, where the vaccine industry would melt into one cohesive glob, reach an

---

[50] "It Just Won't Go Away" Email Thomas Verstraeten to Bob Davis, CDC, Dec. 17, 1999.

agreement, and eschew dissenters by not inviting them as part of the fifty-two experts on the guest list. The CDC's Bob Chen, Frank DeStefano, and Dr. Walter Orenstein (director of NIP) would attend the two-day summit on thimerosal, while the agency's visiting scientist Poul Thorsen and, by then, his paramour, mistress, girlfriend senior epidemiologist Diana Schendel, would stay back at CDC headquarters.

Dr. Coleen Boyle needed to flatten the data, cook it, and filter it to show no causation existed between thimerosal in vaccines and the alarming, rising rates of autism in the United States—the highest in the world—at the turn of the millennium.

But that April, Boyle had little time to get Tom Verstraeten to find a way to recalculate the biostatics of his study. So she did the next best thing. She took the long horizon. In order to eliminate the high impact harm that thimerosal could have on some babies, Dr. Boyle emailed Frank DeStefano outlining the seven bullet points to cure the results. Of the seven, point two showed where she was heading in manipulating the data:

"Since most of the dx's [diagnoses] are generally not picked up until the 2nd or 3rd year of life, had you considered eligibility criteria of at least 18 months or 2 years? What happens if you do this?"[51]

It's obvious what would happen if a coach did that to data on his college football team. The data would get boiled. Ninety players on the roster across all four classes with six red-shirt freshmen quarterbacks. The goal of the data analysis would be to get the optimum size, speed, weight, and strength of the average player on the team. The first run spits out a slow, doughboy-type player. Not good enough. So coach runs the analysis again, this time eliminating the puny, lightweight kicker, punters, and red-shirt freshman. But that

---

[51] "Comments on Analysis" Email Coleen Boyle to Frank DeStefano, CDC, 4-25-2000.

dataset produces a heavier, even slower player. So in the third set, he eliminates all linemen over 300 pounds, weak freshmen, and slow runners of all sizes. When the coach runs the third analysis, the team has been pared down to twenty-nine twenty-nine players. The new dataset produces the ideal player: 6'2" tall, 255 pounds, fast 4.55 speed in the 40–yard dash, and the ability to benchpress 25 reps of 300-pounds.

This data is so sexy to the coach that he tells the marketing team to play with the sizes (height, weight, speed) of the players in the football lineup program to give the impression that his team was loaded with studs and thoroughbreds.

Coleen Boyle took a similar approach to boil the data to achieve the ideal results for her preferred outcome—no link showing any adverse affects on thimerosal.

By showing DeStefano how easy it would be to skew, massage, or manipulate the data, Dr. Boyle set the tone for the secret Simpsonwood meeting to be held in two months. It would be a conference that would pit vaccine policymakers (CDC), vaccine safety (FDA, CDC), and representatives from the pharmaceutical industry. The situation would be akin to the NRA, pro-gun policymakers, the Red Cross, and gun manufacturers meeting at a retreat with a full press blackout and U.S. citizens left in the dark. And those invited agreed ahead of time that semiautomatic, full-mag guns were safe, no matter how many people and children suffered injuries.

Because Poul Thorsen was working on cerebral palsy studies at the time, Boyle prepped Thomas Verstraeten, according to a source, to deliver his findings as is, but to expect those in attendance to take over the conversation.

The secret meeting was held on June 7th and 8th, 2000, at the Simpsonwood Conference Center and Retreat in Norcross, Georgia, twenty-four miles northeast of Atlanta. With "20,000 square feet of meeting space," Tom Verstraeten became the center of attention in the main hall, the focal point of the CDC, FDA, NIH, the WHO, universities, and pharmaceutical representatives. Also in attendance were several doctors and scientists who had attended the aluminum meeting in Puerto Rico one month before.

The notables in attendance were the WHO's John Clements, from Geneva by way of New Zealand; Bob Chen, chief of Vaccine Safety and Development at the National Immunization Program, CDC; and Martin Myers, the acting director of the National Vaccine Program Office. Understanding that aluminum salts as adjuvants in vaccines were not making headline news, while attending the Simpsonwood "Scientific Review of Vaccine Safety Datalink Information" the trio drifted in a fog of a déjà vu of sorts as they would recall the anxious, contested aluminum meeting held the year before in the NIH auditorium in Bethesda.

Joining Chen and Verstraeten from the CDC was Frank DeStefano, project director of the Vaccine Safety Datalink, as well as Jose Cordero, deputy director of NIP, among others.

After listening to the discussion centered on Tom Verstraeten's study, which showed a connection between thimerosal containing vaccines and autism, John Clements grew agitated. Like the New Zealander had done at the aluminum meeting in Puerto Rico a month earlier, Clements calculated the time and the billions of dollars it would cost to remove thimerosal and replace it with another preservative. Worse, he feared, would be the potential fallout of many mothers and fathers in the herd of the vaccinated population losing faith with the program and leaving it in droves. He would let the first day's proceedings and most of the second day roll on. Then he tuned into Tom Verstraeten's exchange with Dr. Robert Brent, a pediatrician and developmental biologist at Thomas Jefferson University and the DuPont Hospital for Children.

"Personally, I have three hypotheses. My first hypothesis is it is parental bias. The children more likely to be vaccinated are more likely to be picked up and diagnosed. Second hypothesis, I don't know. There is a bias that I have not recognized. And nobody has yet told me about it. Third hypothesis, it's true. It's thimerosal. Those are my hypotheses,"[52] Dr. Verstraeten said.

Dr. Brent responded: "If it's true, which or what mechanisms would you explain the finding with?"

"You're asking for biological plausibility?" Verstraeten asked.

"Well, yes,"[53] Brent replied.

From there Dr. Tom Verstraeten wandered about in his answer, discussing the Faroe study, which "looked at PCB." Then he mentioned at animal studies, comparing studies between the Faroe and Seychelles populations, to which he said, on the record, "That means I cannot exclude such a possible effect."[54]

Thimerosal's impact on neurodevelopmental issues in vaccinated babies was squarely put on the table. All John Clements could do at that moment was clench his fist and imagine grasping his hiking stick. Dr. Verstraeten did not stop there. He went on to discuss the "irreversible damage" that thimerosal would do to infants, especially in the first month of being vaccinated. That remark stuck in Clements's craw.

Earlier that day, Dr. Clements recalled what CDC Bob Chen had said: "One of the reasons that led me personally to not be so quick to dismiss the findings was that on his own, Tom independently picked three different outcomes that he did not think could be associated with mercury and three out of three had a different pattern across the different exposure levels as compared to the ones that again on a priority basis, we picked as biologically plausible to be due to mercury exposure."[55]

To which Dr. Brent asked, "Which one of the three that would not be associated with mercury?"

---

[52]  Simpsonwood Transcript, pg. 165, June 7–8, 2000.

[53]  Ibid, pg. 166.

[54]  Ibid, pg. 166.

[55]  Ibid, pg. 151.

Dr. Verstraeten answered, "One was conjunctivitis, diarrhea, and injury."

"Flat feet,"[56] added Dr. Isabelle Rapin, a neurologist for children at Albert Einstein College of Medicine.

If Dr. Clements thought the piling on thimerosal would end there, he was mistaken.

Later on, Dr. Bill Weil, a pediatrician representing the Committee on Environmental Health of the Academy, said, "The number of doses related relationships are linear and statistically significant. You can play with this all you want. They are linear. They are statistically significant." Without mincing words, he said the results of the Verstraeten abstract study showed a clear tie, a relationship that thimerosal was, in fact, a trigger for a series of developmental issues in babies.

Ever the hiker, when John Clements's turn came to speak later that day, he told the rapt audience that he wanted to stand to deliver his message. Like being back in his homeland, navigating the paths, trails, and footfalls over various climbs and hikes up mountains and down slopes into valleys, Clements grasped the opportunity to navigate the mostly American medical audience.

He stood in front of the fifty-one peers at the conference and spoke plainly but with passion, allowing his magnetic presence and his Australian accent to steer his words through their minds, saying, "I am really concerned that we have taken off like a boat going down one arm of the mangrove swamp at high speed when in fact there was not enough discussion really early on about which way the boat should go at all. And I really want to risk offending everyone in the room by saying that perhaps this study should not have been done at all."[57]

The boat lost in a mangrove swamp was a strong image that grabbed the audience right out of the gate. He urged his scientific peers to think, reminding them that handling the thimerosal issue would be "extremely

---

[56] Ibid, pg. 151.
[57] Ibid, pg. 247.

problematic." Feeling that it was too late to reverse course on removing thimerosal, Clements doubled down, stood his ground, and said, "My mandate as I sit here in this group is to make sure at the end of the day that 100,000,000 are immunized with DTP, Hepatitis B, and if possible Hib, this year, next year, and many years to come, and that will have to be with thimerosal-containing vaccines unless a miracle occurs and an alternative is found quickly and is tried and found to be safe."[58]

John Clements finished by reemphasizing his concern that the controversy on thimerosal and vaccines had "gone too far" and that it had to stop. There would be no turning around, no going back, no placating the public. As a group, they would have to come together on messaging the issue.

After listening to the political rhetoric of Dr. Clements and others like him who, in essence, would sweep the thimerosal controversy under the carpet and keep the vaccine immunization program fully intact with more shots and booster shots to come online in the new century, Tom Verstraeten decided to get a second opinion. He went to an expert on metals—lead, mercury—toxicity in fish, children, and the environment in Danish-educated Philippe Grandjean, MD, PhD.

Born in Denmark in 1950 and having earned his MD from University of Copenhagen in 1973 at the age of twenty-three, Dr. Grandjean would offer Verstraeten a fresh outside opinion. When Tom Verstraeten emailed him five weeks after Simpsonwood, he had copied Bob Chen, Frank DeStefano, and four other science experts on vaccines and immunology.

Out of the gate, Verstraeten "apologized for dragging" Philippe Grandjean "into the nitty gritty discussion." He qualified that he did want to "drag the Faroe and Seychelles studies into this entire thimerosal debate."[59]

---

[58] Ibid, pg. 247.

[59] Email from Tom Verstraeten to Philippe Grandjean, July 14, 2000.

Politically sensitive to who paid him, the CDC, and where he would spend the rest of his career (in the pharmaceutical industry with next stop at GlaxoSmithKline Biologics), Tom Verstraeten also said: "I do not want to be the advocate of the anti-vaccine lobby and sound like being convinced that thimerosal is or was harmful, but at least I feel we should use sound scientific argumentation and not let our standards be dictated by our desire to disprove an unpleasant theory."[60]

Dr. Philippe Grandjean, who was a Harvard professor at that time, agreed to look at Verstraeten's questions.

Trying to lead a horse to water to somehow bless that there wasn't enough accurate data to show causation between thimerosal in vaccines and autism, the Belgium doctor took a risk bringing in a Danish world-renowned expert in heavy metals toxicity. In 1979, Grandjean had "defended his doctoral thesis on the 'Widening perspectives of lead toxicity'. He became Professor of Environmental Medicine at the University of Southern Denmark in 1982."[61]

This was a no-nonsense Dane. He stood up to the skeptical establishment and won with his conviction and expertise on environmental causes on neurological and developmental disorders.

Still, in the coming months, at the behest of his CDC peers and superiors, Tom Verstraeten was more concerned about appearances, public scrutiny, and fallout from the false myth that mercury was safe instead of publishing his then year-old abstract as it was and letting the real numbers and linear statistics point to thimerosal as the leading candidate in many infant developmental disorders.

A review of the Verstraeten and DeStefano study by Brian Hooker et al. in 2014, "Methodological Issues and Evidence of Malfeasance in Research Purporting to Show Thimerosal in Vaccines Is Safe," revealed the following salient facts:

---

[60] Ibid.

[61] Biography: http://www.hsph.harvard.edu/philippe-grandjean/

- "This study was conducted in at least five separate phases."[62]
- "In the final phase (i.e., the results reported in the publication), the authors stated that there was no relationship between thimerosal exposure in vaccines and autism incidence. However, no data are reported in the published study to support this conclusion."[63]
- "Using records from (4) HMOs showed that infants who were exposed to greater than 25 μg of Hg in vaccines and immunoglobulins at the age of one month were 7.6 times more likely to have an autism diagnosis than those not exposed to any vaccine-derived organic Hg."[64]
- "Within the same abstract, Verstraeten reports that the risk for any neurodevelopmental disorder was 1.8, the risk for speech disorder was 2.1, and the risk for nonorganic sleep disorder was 5.0. All relative risks were statistically significant."[65]

If these results had been published in 2000 before the Simpsonwood meeting, thimerosal would have been permanently removed from all vaccines then. But had Dr. Maurice heeded the warning coming from Hans Wigzell out of Sweden in 1992 on thimerosal neuro-toxicity instead of keeping Merck's vaccine engine well lubricated in terms of sales and growth; had the 101st Congress two years before gotten President George H. W. Bush to clean out the CDC Agent Orange data manipulators, in particular Dr. Coleen Boyle; had the CDC acted on the letters from the pharmaceutical companies stating they could remove thimerosal from their vaccines; had all of the scientists and doctors who attended the two secret meetings on aluminum and thimerosal done the right thing for the health and welfare of babies and

---

[62] BioMed Research International, Vol. 2014, Article ID 247218, Brian Hooker et al., pg. 4.

[63] Ibid, pg. 4.

[64] Ibid, pg. 4.

[65] Ibid, pg. 5.

their families, then perhaps the explosion in speech delays, body tics, motor impairments, the regressive form of autism, ADHD, ADD, peanut allergies, among other neurological or immunological disorders could have been curbed, if not contained.

The opportunity cost of the vaccine monolith made up of government agencies operating unchecked and unfettered by either the Senate, Congress, or the White House for the past quarter of a century has cost the future of America in terms of lifelong chronic health ailments. On the other side of this double-edge sword, most of those masses of ailing children will not work when they reach adulthood, thus won't be paying taxes into the system, instead becoming drains on families, cities, states, and the federal government.

Having already locked up a cooperative agreement between his newly formed research group out of Aarhus University with the CDC, Poul Thorsen saw the internal desperation, heard the hushed conversations, and felt the tension of CDC executives trying to get ahead of the story. In the thimerosal-autism controversy that wouldn't die down, Thorsen saw how Coleen Boyle in particular and the CDC as a whole operated without impunity. They could do no harm to themselves.

All the CDC had to do was manipulate the data to "prove" thimerosal was safe, that vaccines weren't related in any way to the autism epidemic, and then get far ahead in the messaging. And for Poul Thorsen, he saw a golden opportunity to deliver what the CDC needed.

## 7

# RECRUITING A POLITICAL ANIMAL

When Poul Thorsen needed a dream partner, someone to legiti-mize who he was and his venture to setup a research group within Aarhus University to procure funding from the United States in grant money from the CDC, NIH, and NAAR/Autism Speaks, among other foundations, he knew he had to reach out and recruit a politically savvy, seasoned, and connected mover and shaker.

His top candidate was Ib Terp, a smart, even-keeled tactician, with an impeccable reputation within the Danish government. Ib was per-sonable, sensible, and knew how to navigate the inner workings of the various agencies in the Danish government he came in contact with through the Danish Medical Research Council, a research body he had worked for since the early 1980s. His round face beamed a charming, engaging smile of the W. C. Fields variety. And Ib Terp always dressed for business in suits or blazers and slacks and a match-ing tie.

In late spring 2015, Ib Terp, was mayor of Brøndby Commune, a Danish town of 35,000 residents forty minutes southwest of Copenhagen. For Mayor Terp, 2015 represented his last year in office as he had decided to retire rather than seek reelection for a fourth term in November. But it also was his most volatile, news-making year since becoming mayor in 2005.

First, Terp had to deal with the fallout from the Islamic terrorist who attacked a cartoon summit in Copenhagen, where he shot and killed a Danish filmmaker and wounded three police officers. Able to escape, terrorist Omar El-Hussein went to a Jewish synagogue and killed a volunteer guard before being shot by Danish police.[66]

Omar El-Hussein had lived in Brøndby. There were all kinds of controversies surrounding his burial and the religious rites. But Ib Terp, who had been a member of the Brøndby municipal city council since 1978, told me during an interview that his town is "23 percent ethnic citizens, many who are second and third generation." Deep down, the steadfast mayor would have to become the bridge of peace and reason between the terrorist's culture in Brøndby and an incensed nation of Danes who wanted some form of retribution for the murders of the people and assassination of freedom of speech and expression.

So Mayor Ib Terp stepped forward and took charge. He spoke with the Danish news media, saying, "Regardless of what he has done, he has the right to a burial," and then added he didn't object to El-Hussein's burial taking place in his district, noting "that he hoped the grave 'does not become a site of pilgrimage.'"[67]

The second matter of the year for Terp was less contentious but just as poignant and solemn to the Danish people of Brøndby. The year Terp marked the 70th anniversary of Denmark's liberation from Nazi Germany.

---

[66] "We Lost the Propaganda War: From Twitter to Denmark," James Grundvig, Epoch Times, A11, March 12, 2015.

[67] "Jewish Victim of Copenhagen Shooting Buried" Deutsche Welle, February 18, 2018 (www.DW.com).

At the wreath-laying ceremony at a local church, Ib Terp read from a prepared speech: "Some traditions around the 4th and 5th of May [are] perhaps a little on the decline, but we have chosen to mark the liberation because it still means a lot to many people. Even as those who lived under the occupation become a shrinking occupation, there are still families living with wounds from the occupation, and therefore it is natural to honor the fallen, while preserving the collective memory of the historic events."[68]

When Poul Thorsen's name was brought up during the interview at the mayor's office, he replied, "I don't know him." When I asked again, he shook his head. He, like many other professionals who have dealt with Dr. Poul Thorsen, didn't want to speak about the research scientist on or off the record. They would rather forget about Thorsen, who would one day become a pariah and leave a debris field of used and scorned people who harbor ill will and acrimony that would stretch from the Eastern Seaboard of the United States across the Atlantic, through Ireland, the United Kingdom, Belgium, and up to his roots in Denmark.

Mayor Terp, ever the gentleman, spoke about his past in the Danish Medical Research Council, where he served in the role of administration secretary. He said, "Twenty years ago, Denmark had six research councils; today there are only three research councils."

Naturally, like any politician and civil servant, Ib Terp hit some public turbulence in August 1985. He got caught in a cancer center that never got built or came to fruition in any form. As head of the State's Research Secretariat, he saw the funding troubles coming. The problem began when the "Danish Cancer Society enjoyed increasing returns in the form of increasing charitable donations from the public and wise investment strategies which gave the organization a new power position and a new basis

---

[68] http://www.brondby.dk/Service/Nyheder/2015/05/Broendby-Kommune-markerede-70-aars-dagen-for-Danmarks-Befrielse.aspx

for deciding whether or not the proposed Rockefeller Centre would in fact serve or impair the cancer charity's new role and objective."[69]

But there came an internal "shift in strategy." And when the cancer center was never built, Ib Terp "was quoted in a newspaper article saying that the MRC (Medical Research Council) and the NSRC (Network Startup Research Center) had deliberately and gradually downsized their allocations for cancer research because of the wealth of the Cancer Society."[70]

In August 1985, an article with the title "The State lets civil citizens pay for the fight against cancer" was run in one of the leading Danish newspapers. The article argued that the State did not assume responsibility for finding and financing a solution to the cancer problem, and even though the Cancer Society was experiencing great increases in its income and supposedly paid for more than two thirds of all cancer research projects, it was continuously dependent on voluntary contributions to be able to prevent the country's anti-cancer efforts from collapsing. Both the journalist of the article and the researchers and officials it quoted used the word "State" without always clarifying which agency, council or ministry they were referring to. This made the allegations against the State a bit confusing, as it is unclear to whom they refer. The "State" became an undefined and blurred opponent.

The article brought quotes from Society chairman and Aarhus physician Steen Olsen and the head of management in the State's Research Secretariat, Ib Terp, who agreed that the State—still meaning the State's research councils, the MRC and the NSRC— had gradually downsized its allocations for cancer research, because

---

[69] "The Cancer Center that Never Was: The Organization of Danish Cancer Research 1949-1992," pg. 202, by Marie Louise Conradsen, Copenhagen Business School 1992.

[70] Ibid, pg. 233-34.

of the newfound wealth of the private cancer charity, so that they could support other worthy research projects.[71]

Was there any political fallout from the cancer center that never was? No, not for Ib Terp. He was merely a spoke in the wheel of the project and a smaller cog in the overall system. He would go on to work on other projects for the Medical Research Council until Poul Thorsen came knocking on his door in 1999. Thorsen's credentials were good enough; he had just earned his PhD from Southern Odense University the year before. He had his own network in Statens Serum Institut and Aarhus University Epidemiology Department.

But even so, with what took place less than a decade later, Ib Terp would not speak about his years and role of being an advisor to Poul Thorsen's new research group, the North Atlantic Neuro-Epidemiology Alliances (NANEA). Setup in 1999 with Terp's help Thorsen would use the future mayor of Brøndby in order to procure funding from the Danish Medical Research Council, Aarhus University, and ultimately the sloth fat cats at the Centers for Disease Control.

So entrenched was Poul Thorsen at the CDC by the turn of the millennium that he had secured his own CDC government email address—not bad for a foreign scientist. When I told one of Thorsen's Danish research scientists that "I, as an American citizen, could never get a CDC email address," the scientist just laughed at the absurdity of it all, especially in light of the actions Poul Thorsen would carry out and perpetrate against the U.S. health agency. It was an agency that would support him, steer his research toward cerebral palsy and autism—two of the emerging red-hot issues in the 21st century— give the young scientist name recognition and thus clout within certain scientific circles, and bestow upon him a seemingly bottomless well of funding. All Thorsen had to do was perform, play the game

---

[71] Ibid, pg. 205.

right, and show gratitude toward the CDC and the pharmacological industry monolith that would shield him from the outside world.

For Poul Thorsen, opening a CDC Credit Union Bank account in Atlanta became part of that team-building effort by the agency. But it would be Ib Terp's name and signature, on behalf of Poul Thorsen and NANEA for which Terp was listed as a "principal investigator" even though he was not a scientist, on the first of two cooperative agreements between the foreign health concern and CDC late in 1999 that got Thorsen rolling. His budding relationship with Diana Schendel would be the icing on a grand cake for a man with a scent for capitalism and a grand vision of research science.

So it is interesting to look back at the career of Ib Terp, armed with a masters of science in chemical engineering from the Technical University of Denmark in 1970, which he would never fully use, as he shifted gears out of a career in the industrial world to become a civil servant and serve the people of Denmark.

Poul Thorsen was all set to serve himself.

By the time fall 2004 came around, Thorsen himself would sign the second cooperative agreement with the CDC since he no longer needed Ib Terp's name to secure funding. Soon he would be awash in CDC capital. He had tapped into the golden vein, a mother lode, by preying on the agency's urgent need to squash some bad information. In order to do that, Dr. Coleen Boyle and her colleagues set out to find promising data.

She had just the right woman in mind to do it.

8

# 2001: A DATA ODYSSEY

As Drs. Tom Verstraeten and Frank DeStefano massaged the data in their thimerosal study for more than a year, the pressure was mounting enough in the court of public opinion that the CDC had to produce a new study on a separate track. That study, to be done in parallel with Verstraeten's, had to be fast tracked on top of showing there was no link between thimerosal containing vaccines and the rising rate of autism.

Coleen Boyle had gone through this drill before with Diana Schendel in 2000. In an email sent one week before the Simpson meeting, Dr. Marshalyn Yeargin-Allsopp wrote to Dr. Jose Cordero, soon to be the first director of the National Birth Defects and Developmental Disabilities in April 2001.[72]

She opened:

As we discussed on Friday, we have become aware through Poul Thorsen of an exciting opportunity to study the role of MMR

---

[72] http://www.cdc.gov/ncbddd/aboutus/timeline/timeline-interactive.html – 2001

vaccine and autism using several registries/existing studies and
the repository of biologic specimens and laboratory capabilities
in Denmark.[73]

Dr. Yeargin-Allsopp attached a budget proposal from Poul
Thorsen's research group NANEA at Aarhus University, in concert
with Ib Terp at the Danish Medical Research Council, about the new
"exciting opportunity." Marshalyn stated that the new NCBDDD
didn't have the funds, so CDC/NIP were the likely candidates to
finance it; Cordero worked at NIP. That meant the CDC now had
a partner that could backtest MMR historical data to produce its
desired results.

But which country outside the U.S. boasted the best databases on
the health of its citizens and had removed thimerosal from vaccines,
like Denmark, Japan, and Sweden did in or around 1992?

One year later in the summer of 2001, the CDC turned to a new
fixer in Dr. Diane M. Simpson, deputy director of the NIP—Jose
Cordero's previous role. A diminutive, middle-aged white woman
with dyed light brown hair hiding the gray that had begun to creep in
over the years, Dr. Simpson not only had to identify that country, but
she also had to beat the clock.

By summer 2001, word had spread that the Institute of Medicine's
(IOM) Immunization Safety Review Committee, would pub-
lish its 136-page report in October called "Immunization Safety
Review: Thimerosal Containing Vaccines and Neurodevelopmental
Disorders." That didn't give Dr. Simpson a big window in which to
achieve her objectives.

Diane Simpson got the ball rolling in June 2001. She emailed
Marshalyn Yeargin-Allsopp, MD, a big boned black woman with
a bright, vivacious smile and wavy, shoulder-length hair. Dr.

---

[73] Email: From Dr. Marshalyn Yeargin-Allsopp to Jose Cordero, "Proposal for
Study of MMR Vaccine and Autism in Denmark" (May 30, 2001).

Yeargin-Allsopp was the chief of Developmental Disabilities Branch, National Center on Birth Defects and Developmental Disabilities (NCBDDD).

Diane Simpson reminded Dr. Yeargin-Allsopp they had met two weeks earlier at the National Vaccine Advisory Committing (NVAC) meeting on May 24. The meeting centered on "NVAC seeks public comments on vaccine financing." In reality it was a NVAC work group for the introduction of new vaccines. Those in attendance could comment on the new shots but more importantly focus on removing the barriers to market entry in rolling out new vaccines. Beyond the funding and trials, the real barriers to entry would be negative press against thimerosal in new vaccines.

The U.S. Department of Health and Human Services (HHS) initially founded NVAC in 1987 to be a lobby-free think tank. And it worked that way until a decade later when the MMR-thimerosal-autism nexus intersected in the American consciousness that vaccines might very well be the underlying cause of the autism epidemic. Thus, at the turn of the millennium, much like the secret offshore aluminum meeting and the even more secretive thimerosal-Simpsonwood meeting, NVAC morphed into a covert cabal to take action to ensure vaccine production, rollout, and sales would run uninterrupted deep into the new century.

After the opening line of the email, Simpson asked for Dr. Yeargin-Allsopp's help: "Can you please tell me who is the best person to talk to in order to get data on autism rates in Denmark? In particular, I am interested in knowing if they reported cases have dramatically increased over the past 10 years as the have in the U.S."[74]

Simpson's next paragraph got to the heart of the matter: "You also mentioned that Denmark has never used thimerosal as a preservative

---

[74] Email June 8, 2001: CDC Diane Simpson to Marshalyn Yeargin-Allsopp.

in their vaccines, but I can't remember if you told me if you were certain of that fact or if I needed to verify it. Are you certain?"[75]

Three hours later, Marshalyn Yeargin-Allsopp responded: "Dr. Diana Schendel who is the PI on our study and is in Denmark this week. Can put you in touch with our contacts in Denmark. You can ask me again, but I am certain about the thimerosal issue."[76]

Diana Schendel was indeed in Denmark that week. In fact, she was with Poul Thorsen, who was showing her around the Aarhus University campus, a ten-minute car ride from the train station up the hilly, idyllic city with a canal that cuts through the center of town. A source at the CDC confirmed that Poul Thorsen was also showing Diana Schendel around the beautiful beaches of Aarhus east of the city center. The working vacation gave the new lovers time for some rest and relaxation as their relationship bloomed that summer.

On June 11, Diane Simpson emailed Autism-Europe asking for "the incidence rate of autism in various European countries." She narrowed her request to the past "10-20 years" with interest in Denmark and Sweden, as she learned that both countries had removed thimerosal from their vaccine schedules, based on Swedish researcher Hans Wigzell's study of the mercury-based preservative and childhood neuro-development issues, such as tics and speech delays.

"Autism-Europe is a European association whose main objective is to advance the rights of people with autism and their families, and help improve their lives."[77]

The organization was based in Brussels, Belgium.

Internally on the same day, Dr. Simpson received information on the vaccine "DTP Coverage and Autism Caseload on Calif – Time Trend Data." The data was presented by year with percentage of

---

[75] Email June 8, 2001: CDC Diane Simpson to Marshalyn Yeargin-Allsopp

[76] Ibid.

[77] *Home Educating Our Autistic Spectrum Children: Paths are Made by Walking*, Edited by Terri Dowty, Kitt Cowlishaw, Pg. 289.

children receiving four (4) doses of DTP shot by the age of two years, and the number of autism cases for each year.

Looking over the fifteen-year period from 1980 to 1994, the coverage went from 50.9% with 176 autism cases in 1980, to 48.9% with 246 cases five years later. By 1990, the coverage increased to 65.9%, while the number of autism cases nearly tripled to 663. In 1994, the coverage exceeded 75% with 1,182 cases. California, like the rest of the United States, had a direct correlation that any child with a straightedge and basic knowledge of Occam's razor principle or Pythagoras's first theorem—that the shortest distance between two points is a straight line—could see as DTP coverage increased, over the number of autism cases soared by 670% over the same time period.[78]

Loring Dales, MD, of the Immunization Branch of California Dept. of Health Services, provided Dr. Simpson with the historical data.

In pulling the pieces of information in from Scandinavia, California, and soon Japan, Diane Simpson was preparing to make a recommendation on what country the CDC should backtest data on that had vaccines that were thimerosal-free. California was out with its fully loaded TCV immunization jabs.

Simpson wrote to Marta Granstrom, M.D., PhD, professor at the Dept. of Clinical Microbiology, Karolinska Hospital, Sweden, titling the email "Vaccine Preservatives":

Has Sweden used thimerosol [sic] (or other mercury containing compounds) as a preservative in their vaccines? If Sweden no longer uses thimerosol [sic] (or a similar compound) do you know when the practice was discontinued?

If you have similar data regarding vaccines used in Denmark, that would also be very helpful.

As an introduction: I am the acting Deputy Director for the National Immunization Program (Dr. Jose Cordero, the previous

---

[78] Email June 8, 2001: Loring Dales, California DHS to CDC Diane Simpson.

deputy director has taken a temporary assignment as head of the CDC's new center on birth defects and developmental disabilities). As you may be aware the use of thimerosol [sic] as a preservative in vaccines has been a source of recent concern. U.S. manufacturers have discontinued its use as a preservative in vaccine products given to young children. I appreciate any information you can provide.[79]

Dr. Granstrom wrote back, responding in a way that must have given Diane Simpson heartburn, if not pause. For Marta Granstrom was no fan of thimerosal, and she clearly overlooked Simpson's inability to spell "thimerosal" correctly, maybe because the Swedish MD and PhD couldn't spell it herself—at least in an unedited email.

What that really meant was Dr. Simpson had never read Hans Wigzell's 1990 brief, "Difficult to Substitute Mercury as a Preservative in Bacterial Vaccines."

"Dear Diane,

"It is correct that Sweden has not used pediatric vaccines containing thiomersal, for many years now—officially it was abandoned in 1989 but since the stock-remaining wgs [sic] sold out, the Swedish Medical Products Agency claims that we should count pediatric vaccines as thiomersal-free [sic] since 1992.

"I know that also Denmark has abandoned the use of thiomersal quite some time ago but I don't know when. I would propose that you contact Michael Stellfeld at the Danish Serum institute (SSI) to get a precise date.

"I am very well aware of the recent concerns in the US over thiomersal. On the expert committee (Group 15 for Vaccines and Sera) of the European Pharmacopoeae I represent Sweden and had in vain tried to get Europe to ban its use in single dose vials until the US interest in the issue (it is removed also from multidose vials in Sweden

---

[79] Email June 8, 2001: CDC Diane Simpson to Marta Granstrom, Sweden.

but that might have been too much to aim for in a first step). In the latest version of the monography of the EU Ph on "Vaccines for Human Use" it now states that single dose vials should not contain a preservative - without the 10 line exceptions that used to follow the statement. I thanked Neal Halsey in the name of European infants for the help when I met him again last year.[80]

This had to be a stunning rebuke for Diane Simpson and the CDC. But like a Colorado-stoned bison in a china shop, instead of taking the warning from Dr. Granstrom, combined with Dr. Tom Verstraeten's 2000 "It Just Won't Go Away" findings, plus the pair of 1999 letters from vaccine manufacturers Merck and GlaxoSmithKline, and other ancillary evidence that piled up like cars at a demolition derby that showed a clear link between thimerosal and spiking autism rates, Simpson and the CDC soldiered on as if none of the other professional insights didn't matter or exist.

Dr. Diane Simpson, with the Centers for Disease Control's blessing, scratched Sweden off the shrinking short list of countries that would give her what she was tasked to find: rising autism rates versus thimerosal-free vaccines.

Who would play ball with Diane Simpson?

She went back to Denmark and her email ten days earlier with Kreesten Meldgaard Madsen, a research scientist and soon-to-be PhD candidate at the university. The way forward for Simpson now resided in Denmark, courtesy of CDC Dr. Diana Schendel via Poul Thorsen and his Aarhus University research group NANEA. The lovers, most likely locked in each other's arms at the time of the email titled "Autism Data," has Simpson reaching out to Madsen:

"Your name was given to me by our new Center for Birth Defects and Developmental Disabilities. I am the acting deputy for the National Immunization Program and need to find whatever data may exist on autism rates in children in Denmark over the last 20 years. As

---

[80]  Email June 22, 2001: Marta Granstrom, Sweden, to CDC Diane Simpson.

always, I need the data sooner rather than later. Any assistance you can provide would be greatly appreciated."[81]

Kreesten Madsen must have smiled at the opportunity, coming from the CDC in wealthy America. They needed his, NANEA's, and Aarhus University's assistance.

Little would Diana Simpson know that her email to Kreesten Madsen would set off a long-acting chain of events that would lead to more twists and turns and bends in the Poul Thorsen saga than can be found in the Mississippi River.

Two weeks later in an email to CDC's Bob Chen, Diane Simpson not only knew how to finally spell "thimerosal" correctly, but also the amount of the preservative in the DTP/Hib vaccine—"50 micrograms thimerosal per dose so that our children would if on schedule have 75 micrograms of ethyl hg by 4 months of age."[82]

Like many managers in different government agencies, the bureaucratic process dropped a new hot project in Simpson's lap. Unfamiliar with the details, such as the new word added to her lexicon in "thimerosal," Diane Simpson dove in head first, reaching out across the globe to pull in the experts she would need to get the tasks done as quickly as possible.

What she didn't likely know, however, was the amount of thimerosal that the birth-shot of Hepatitis B vaccine contained or how the immunization was approved.

From the government's "The Pink Sheet" of June 4, 1984, an in depth efficacy report on vaccines, the "Text" reads:

Merck's <r> DNA-produced Hepatitis B Vaccine Effectiveness in Humans in a clinical trial conducted by the company was

---

[81] Email June 12, 2001: CDC Diane Simpson to Kreesten M. Madsen, Aarhus University Dept. of Epidemiology.

[82] Email June 25, 2001: CDC Diane Simpson to Bob Chen "UK Vaccine Schedule and Thimerosal Exposure."

reported in June 1 JAMA. 'The results of this study indicate that an alum-absorbed hepatitis B vaccine formulated using hepatitis B surface antigen (HBsAg) of subtype adw synthesized by recombinant yeast cells is safe and immunogenic for man,' the Merck researchers reported.[83]

Two problems jump off the first paragraph of this Pink Sheet. First, Merck tested and thus essentially approved its own vaccine for "safety and efficacy" by Merck researchers. Second, the tests were "safe and immunogenic for man," not babies, infants, toddlers, children or even teenagers. Immunogenic simply means to be able to produce an "immune response" to a disease.

The next paragraph from the Pink Sheet gets to the heart of the issue:

The study was conducted among 37 healthy, low-risk adult Merck employees who were vaccinated with a 10-ug dose of HBsAg at 0, 1 and 6 months. The subjects were divided into two groups, 15 of which received vaccine purified by the immune affinity chromatography method, and 22 by the hydrophobic intraction chromatography method.[84]

Only "37 healthy, low-risk adult Merck employees." What does that mean? Were the 37 Merck employees in their 20s and 30s— already vaccinated from the 1950-60s era they were born? Were they top athletes within Merck? Were they all men? Women? A mix to make Hepatitis B safe "for man"? The 1984 Super Bowl Champion San Francisco 49ers had forty-four "healthy, low-risk adults" on its starting offensive and defensive teams.

---

[83] 1984 F-D-C Reports, Inc., "The Pink Sheet" 46 (23) : T&G-3, June 4, 1984, Length: 427 words.

[84] Ibid.

Without third party quality control and quality assurance in place to test the efficacy and safety of a vaccine manufacturer's next concoction in a clinical trial, which didn't mimic real world conditions for a baby being born (0 month), breastfeeding (1 month), and crawling (6 month) in weights that range from 6 to 21 pounds, how does an adult 100 to 250 pounds correlate with that of a baby?

Making matters worse, two years later Merck's Hepatitis B vaccine "was approved by the FDA on July 23, (1986), within five months of the submission of a license application, and within seven years from the time of the initial characterization of the hepatitis B virus gene"[85] by none other than Dr. Maurice Hilleman.

In the mid 1980s, with no mobile phones, no ability to surf the World Wide Web, and no email per se, Merck was able to get the FDA to sign-off on a baby vaccine in five-short months using a clinical trial of a handful of its own adult employees who, by the way, were "healthy" and "low-risk." In the latter, that could have meant they were non-alcoholics, non-diabetes sufferers, had strong hearts, and were non-smokers, and the like. Merck's adult employees might not have been able to cover the 49ers passing attack of 1984, but then they don't have to; all they had to do was take shots on behalf of babies for the betterment of mankind, but Merck's bottom line, receiving the full blessing of the FDA and CDC ever since.

---

[85] 1986 F-D-C Reports, Inc., "The Pink Sheet" 48 (30) : 3-4, July 28, 1986, Length: 1,070 words

# PART II

# THE CULT OF VAINGLORY

# 9

# SLEEPING WITH THE "FRENEMY"

On a sunny Monday in June 2015, I met Palle Valentiner-Branth, MD, PhD, on the century-old campus of Statens Serum Institut (SSI) in central Copenhagen. As head of Vaccine Production and MRSA Group, Department of Infectious Disease Epidemiology, Division of National Health Surveillance & Research, the slender, graying scientist took me on a tour of the old army barracks that have been converted to modern offices.

Adjusting his wire-rimmed glasses, Dr. Valentiner-Branth, who spent nine years on infectious disease and vaccine research in Nepal, told the story of how the land we stood on—today a garden and parking lot—was once a barn with stables and a farm for horses to roam. In 1902, Danish doctors worked with horse, cow, and sheep blood serum to learn more about blood cells, antibodies, and how vaccines could help humans build immunity against certain infectious diseases. That same year, Denmark created Statens Serum Institut to continue that original work.

Since its early beginnings, SSI became the country's state-run manufacturer of vaccines, as well as the monitor of vaccine surveillance—sort of like what Merck was able to do and get away with in the 1980s with its Hepatitis B vaccine. That double duty, ridden with conflicts of interest and with little more than a building separating the producer from the quality assurance monitor, has worked better than the monolith of CDC-FDA-IOM-NIH and their sub-agencies fused to the pharmaceutical industry, with no wall separating big pharma from former agency executives, such as the one-time director of the CDC, Dr. Julie Louise Gerberding, who today works as president of Merck's Vaccine Division.

The most eye-opening line that Dr. Palle Valentiner-Branth delivered was when he said, "Denmark's vaccine schedule starts when a baby is three months old. There is no birth shot. Denmark only vaccinates for nine diseases in boys and ten diseases in girls."

In comparison to the United States, Denmark has a very sane and clean vaccine schedule. It takes Socrates's "less is more" approach on the quantity, components, timing, and spacing of its vaccines, and it hasn't included thimerosal since 1992, when the shelf stock ran out.

"One day soon, we will remove the polio vaccine" from our schedule, since the polio disease is all but eradicated," Dr. Valentiner-Branth said.

When Denmark does remove the polio vaccine from its schedule, will the CDC follow suit and remove the polio jab from the U.S. immunization schedule? Or, because polio vaccines with all its boosters make far too much money for the pharmaceutical industry, will the CDC refuse to do it? Or will the CDC delay the removal several years beyond one projected eradication date of 2018. The WHO's "the new Polio Eradication and Endgame Strategic Plan, released on April 11, 2013, and developed by the (WHO's) Global Polio Eradication Initiative, has committed signatories to eradicate polio by 2018."[86]

Is it be hard to imagine the monolith of the CDC allowing the polio vaccine to be dropped from the childhood vaccine schedule

---

[86] The Disease Daily: http://www.healthmap.org/site/diseasedaily/article/polio-be-eradicated-2018-41213

in order not to disrupt the revenue stream to the bottom line of the giant multinational corporations and not be replaced by a new mandatory vaccine or two?

For Diane Simpson, had she calculated the DTP/Hib bioaccumulation of ethylmercury in a Danish infant's body, she would have arrived at no thimerosal, as in 0.0 micrograms enter a baby, infant or child at any point in their life. Moreover, a Danish baby doesn't receive its first vaccine until the age of three months. There is no Hepatitis B vaccine at birth of a newborn, probably because even though that child wouldn't be exposed to the communicable disease transmission from sex or sharing needles with drug users for another dozen years or more.

Nevertheless, the CDC and FDA continue to insist that the clinical trial of "Hep B" is needed for babies, when in fact those infants wouldn't be exposed to the disease until their teenage years. So it brings into question the efficacy and safety of Hep B, and whether the vaccine is needed at all, or is simply a moneymaker for Big Pharma.

If vaccines are finally proven to be the cause behind the skyrocketing rates of the regressive form of autism, then the tsunami of the neurological disorder in the 21st century starts with Merck's "money shot," fast-tracked by the FDA, with zero third party quality control or quality assurance, and blessed by the CDC on the day the baby is born.

Happy birthday!

Jab!

Welcome to the world!

You now are more likely to get tics, speech delays, and some form of autism than your grandparents, who never received the birth shot of Hepatitis B.

While Diane Simpson continued her odyssey to search for good data to support the CDC's position that mercury is safe to inject into babies, Bob Chen reached out to the vaccine authorities in the

United Kingdom. In essence, the UK used nearly the same amount of thimerosal in its vaccine program as the United States. Dr. Chen, who attended both the secret aluminum meeting in Puerto Rico and the thimerosal Simpsonwood meeting north of Atlanta, was working with a group of international scientists on a project called the Brighton Collaboration, so named after the British coastal town made famous by Graham Greene's 1938 novel *Brighton Rock* for the hard rock-candy found at the summer retreat.

The confectionary candy was Greene's metaphor for man's character under fire in the murder thriller, and it could very well be repurposed as a metaphor for the monolith of the CDC, serving no one but the interests of big industry and other government agencies, which were bought off a long time ago.

In 2000, the non-profit Brighton Collaboration was a voluntary organization founded on the premise of being "an independent global vaccine safety research network for healthcare professionals."[87]

In the Digital Age, the Brighton Collaboration would leverage the Internet, mine databases, and share data "to facilitate the development, evaluation, and dissemination of high quality information about the safety of human vaccines. The idea of the collaboration started in 1999, following a presentation by Dr. Bob Chen at an international scientific vaccine conference in Brighton, U.K. In his talk, he stressed the need to improve vaccine safety monitoring by developing internationally accepted standards."[88]

Whose standards would those be? Denmark? The United States? Or other?

The Brighton Collaboration's conceit on "vaccine safety" and "developing internationally accepted standards," is at bare minimum both false and tone deaf, if not an out and out howler.

---

[87] https://en.wikipedia.org/wiki/Brighton_Collaboration
[88] Ibid.

In August 2002, Jan Bonhoeffer, University Children's Hospital Basel, Basel, Switzerland, together with Bob Chen and seven other scientists wrote the paper, "The Brighton Collaboration: addressing the need for standardized case definitions of adverse events following immunization (AEFI)," published in Vaccine/Elsevier.

It opens with the patently false screamer: "In keeping with the Hippocratic oath, 'First Do No Harm,' any medical intervention including vaccines should be shown safe and effective prior to widespread adoption."[89]

Really? The United States, thanks to the CDC and FDA and others in power of its over-the-top, misguided vaccine program, has done plenty of harm. They have done more harm in the ensuing years by trying to cover up their Hansel and Gretel breadcrumbs with the CDC's empty, tin-car national tour of "Autism Listening Sessions."

The tragic comedy would be even funnier if it didn't include the lives of more than one million damaged U.S. children on the spectrum. The reality is that opening statement can never be achieved until the FDA mandates real clinical trials of vaccines with real saline placebos on its intended audience—infants under three months of age. And that means conducting new independent trials on real babies all over again for Merck's Hepatitis B shot.

Any volunteers?

No. Certainly not a single parent at Merck, CDC, FDA or NIH today would allow their children or grandchildren to go through such a Shirley Jackson-type lottery—in which each year a village randomly selects and stones to death a citizen—that real clinical trials would require. And not the backtesting of data, by way of Denmark, which can be manipulated one hundred different ways.

---

[89] "The Brighton Collaboration: addressing the need for standardized case definitions of adverse events following immunization (AEFI)," J. Bonhoeffer, et. al., Elsevier, Vaccine 21 2002, pg. 298.

On November 22, 2012, before the US House of Representatives, CDC's Coleen Boyle gave testimony on vaccines, birth defects, and what the CDC was doing about it at that time in the wake of the Poul Thorsen scandal.

Not satisfied with her prepared, political-cover statement, U.S. Congressman Bill Posey (8th District, R–FL) called Dr. Coleen Boyle "evasive" and asked her point blank: "Have you done a study comparing autism rates in vaccinated and unvaccinated children?" Unable to answer the question directly, she danced around the question. "After she wasted three minutes, I cut her off and I demanded that she answer the question," Congressman Posey recounted the story for a radio show in April 2014. "And then, only then, did she admit that the federal government has never done that very simple, fundamental, basic study."[90]

In fact, no country or health agency in the world has ever attempted, let alone conducted that kind of clinical trial—not even Merck on the babies of its own employees.

So as CDC's Bob Chen has long pretended to be part of the solution on vaccine safety, he has hidden in the open and become a conduit for the CDC on vaccine intelligence, pulling intel from an array of international scientists and sources. Was Bob Chen a spy? No, not in the Cold War sense of the word. But clearly, Dr. Chen was a CDC scout.

If the Brighton Collaboration's main objective was to standardize vaccine safety, why hasn't the United States banned thimerosal from all vaccines fifteen years after the Collaboration's founding? Why hasn't it eliminated the unnecessary birth-day Hep B shot, and lessen the fourteen vaccines with 69 components to match Denmark's safer—and lower autism rate by a factor of ten—immunization schedule?

Salient facts are hard to disguise. Spin, talking heads, and messaging have long been the arrows in the CDC quiver, dating back to the Agent

---

[90] http://nsnbc.me/2014/04/17/congressman-blasts-cdc-incestuous-relationships-vaccine-makers/

Orange cover-up studies. It goes back to what Dr. Max Lum told the rapt audience of scientists, epidemiologists, and aluminum experts at the Puerto Rico aluminum meeting: "Control the message. It's all about positioning the message."

By any standard, the Brighton Collaboration has failed its mission. And that became more evident in the "Conclusion" of their paper, which reads: "Diversity in safety methods leads to considerable loss of scientific information."[91]

What does that gobbledygook mean? Were these vaccine scientists turned into astrophysicists referring to an event horizon on the rim of a black hole, when all forms of matter, atoms, and molecules spaghettified in a singularity? Has a line ever been more broad, vague, and designed to blame vaccine safety all at the same time? And if the Brighton Collaboration couldn't agree on "safety methods," then what did it expect to accomplish? Blame safety? Discover there are too many diverse methods on safety?

And those "volunteers" represent the gatekeepers of a needle laden with thimerosal or an inactivated virus, and other cool stuff like human, bovine, and sheep DNA, three kinds of aluminum adjuvants, and much, much more.

It appears the Collaboration would share nothing more than information. Not a single nation the founding volunteers represented changed anything in their own country's existing vaccine program other than looking for new ways to help big pharma add more vaccines to a nation's immunization schedules.

The next sentence of the conclusion: "We have built the necessary international network of currently about 300 participants from patient care, public health, scientific, pharmaceutical, regulatory and

---

[91] "The Brighton Collaboration: addressing the need for standardized case definitions of adverse events following immunization (AEFI)," J. Bonhoeffer, et. al., Elsevier, Vaccine 21 2002, pg. 298.

professional organizations to develop and assess standardized AEFI case definitions and guidelines."[92]

The Collaboration's "300" is not to be confused with Sparta's epic and heroic "300" warriors who defended their home from tens of thousands of marauding Persian raiders some 2,500 years ago. Since its inception, the Brighton Collaboration had accomplished little more than building a deep pool of science specialists who shared what they learned and what they discovered in their hospitals, universities, and research labs back home. The sharing of specialized ideas, like Bob Chen's, has been happening since the hunter-gathers turned into farmers some 8,000 years ago, domesticating animals and farming along the way.

For Diane Simpson and her CDC colleagues who worked on her special project of identifying the right country to backtest, the TCVs would drag through July 2001 since many people around the world went on summer holiday, including herself. When she returned to CDC headquarters in the first week of August, she realized then the CDC couldn't possibly do a study on time to meet the IOM October report date.

Although she sent out a flurry of emails on Monday, August 6, 2001, two emails stood out in her search for favorable data with a friendly partner who would play ball. At 1:12 pm, Diane Simpson sent an email to Jeanette and Paul Stehr-Green, the latter an attendee at the Simpsonwood meeting a year earlier. At the time, Paul Stehr-Green was an epidemiologist in training and an associate professor of epidemiology at the University of Washington School of Public Health and Community Medicine. Fourteen months after Simpsonwood, it appeared that Stehr-Green had kicked off his training wheels as an epidemiologist.

With misspellings of the Danish name Poul (not "Paul") and Kreesten (not "Christian"), Diane Simpson was trying to confirm

[92] Ibid.

whether Poul Thorsen was still in Denmark and that she would try to connect with Kreesten Madsen. She also wanted to confirm who "the CDC person assigned to Denmark" was and that she was setting up a conference call to accelerate selecting that country and team. She also mentioned that Diana Schendel was going to contact another Danish scientist.

The thread of that email began on the Thursday before, August 2nd. In her initial email "Charts" to Paul Stehr-Greene, Simpson wrote:

A few things have happened this morning regarding data from Denmark.

I spoke this morning with Diana Schendel in the Center for Birth Defects and Developmental Disabilities (NCBDDD) who is associated with the study of MMR and autism that NCBDDD is conducting in Denmark. The person they Have working in Denmark on the MMR-autism study is Christian [sic] _____ (didn't get the last name). . . .

Persons within NCBDDD have seen the autism data from the registry (and have helped cleared up some coding problems) but evidently feel they cannot share it with us at NIP without the permission of Preben-Bo who has said "no" release before he publishes. However, in my conversation with Diana this morning, I have re-emphasized that we may only need to see/use a small piece of the overall data set or could even discuss with the researcher other (less desirable) possibilities such as making general statements about trends with the actual data being released later.[93]

Simpson's email rambles on, misspelling Madsen's first name again. Now that she could spell thimerosal correctly, the deputy director at

---

[93] Email: From CDC Diane Simpson to CDC Paul Stehr-Green, "Charts," August 2, 2001.

NIP asked Stehr-Green to let her—thus, the CDC, the study's sponsor—to share inside information before the results of the study had reached a natural conclusion. That had happened with the Verstraeten thimerosal study, too. It was happening all over again. Why? Why would the sponsor of a study want to stick its nose out and prematurely find out the results of a study unless it wanted to build a message or control fallout with it, or redo the study a new way in order to flatten or erase any negative findings or correlation that did fit its storyline?

So, as with the new Madsen MMR Study, data would be manipulated as was being done with the Tom Verstraeten thimerosal study. Since Sweden was no longer a viable option with Dr. Marta Granstrom clearly against preservatives even in single dose vials, Diane Simpson would turn toward Denmark for the next round with Kreesten Madsen as principal investigator on his own thimerosal study.

Paul Stehr-Green replied to Simpson's email in an overly friendly tone:

"Man, you lead an exciting life (or maybe just fast-moving)!!

"Thanks for the update and the charts (although I'm even less convinced of a possible association after seeing them). I'll be there all day, so call or email if you hear more and want me to join you. Take care. Paul"[94]

Paul Stehr-Green and Diane Simpson resolved to make the conference call happen. One hour later at 2:54 pm, Paul Stehr-Green wrote:

"What, if anything, are we going to do about getting data from other countries—e.g., Japan, Australia, New Zealand, others? Specifically, are we planning to send team(s) to any other places to consult with local investigators and collect other relevant data?"[95]

Three hours later, Diane Simpson wrote back all but giving up, for the moment, to either find the answer or even "think about it." She seemed exhausted by the logistics and the many potential avenues to

---

[94] Email: From Paul Stehr-Greene to Diane Simpson, "Ongoing Investigation of Thimerosal" August 6, 2001.

[95] Ibid.

search for the right data in other countries, including how the data was gathered, collated, disseminated, and coded to where the CDC scientists could understand whether that local data would be useful or not.

On Tuesday, August 7, Diane Simpson emailed Swedish pediatrician, Christopher Gillberg, with the subject line "Autism Data in Sweden." She wrote: "The US does not have a system to routinely capture data on cases of autism. . . . I also believe that you have conducted surveys for autism over time in a specific area in Sweden. We would be very interested in speaking to you or your colleagues about the data you have."[96]

In a separate email on the same day, Simpson wrote:

"I don't have any new data at the moment and am frantically trying to see what is available and how best to get it in time for the expected IOM report release (we have given up trying to submit it in time for the report as they are in the process of writing it)."

By the next day, Dr. Diane Simpson took charge in an email, talking about "setting something up in the very near future" and discussing the directions of the analyses with the likes of Dr. William Thompson. Bob Chen was cc'd on the email.

Dr. Walter Orenstein, director of the National Immunization Program and the moderator of the Simpsonwood meeting, confirmed for Diane Simpson that she and Paul Stehr-Green would travel together to Denmark on August 22, 2001, and return a week later. His intention was clear. Knowing that Kreesten Madsen and Poul Thorsen were deeply immersed in doing the debunking MMR Study on behalf of the CDC, it would only be natural for his NIP deputy to meet the principal investigator, Dr. Madsen, and the thimerosal study coordinator, Dr. Thorsen, so she could feel out, if they were capable, if they would play ball, and how fast they could turn around

---

[96] Email 8-7-2001: From CDC Diane Simpson to Christopher Gillberg, "Autism Data in Sweden."

to complete such a backtested cohort study from the Danish Health Registries.[97]

The trip to Denmark was a success. When Diane Simpson returned with her findings, which clearly showed that the thimerosal study should be conducted in Denmark with Poul Thorsen's team, it was already the week of Labor Day, which fell early that year on September 3.

Like her peers, colleagues, and partners inside and out of the CDC, Dr. Diane Simpson would have no idea on how the events of Tuesday, September 11, 2001, would impact her life, the course of the CDC, and the need for the newly elected President George W. Bush to mold the future of the leading U.S. health agency.

But as the saying goes, the more things change, the more they would stay the same. The CDC as big pharma monolith would get stronger, and head executives, like Drs. Julie Louis Gerberding and Coleen Boyle, would improve their career and political body armor from Kevlar to Teflon.

Osama bin Laden's al-Qaeda-sponsored terrorist attacks on New York City's World Trade Center and the Beltway's Pentagon all but cemented the political might of the Centers for Disease Control.

---

[97] Email Aug. 6, 2001: From CDC Diane Simpson to Jeanette and Paul Stehr-Green.

# I 0

# THE GOLDEN GIRL OF BIOTERRORISM

After Diane Simpson and Paul Stehr-Green had returned from Denmark, assured that the Scandinavian country was the right place to conduct backtested studies using the Danish Health Registries as a national cohort that had a thimerosal-free immunization schedule against a rise in autism rates, a global event that would change the course of history in the new millennium would also change the direction of the CDC.

September 11, 2001.

On a "severe" clear, blue Tuesday morning, nineteen al-Qaeda terrorists hijacked four planes with little more than box-cutters. Instead of flying the planes to a remote location to make demands for the release of the hostages—the 20th century model—the first plane smashed into the North Tower of the World Trade Center in downtown New York City. Seventeen minutes later, the next jet sliced into the upper floors of the South Tower. Eventually, a third stolen jet slammed into the Pentagon when the hijackers couldn't locate the Capitol Building on the ground after taking over the cockpit. Fortunately for those who lived in densely populated Washington, DC, the fourth jet, Flight

93, crashed into a field in western Pennsylvania, killing all on board rather than anyone at its intended target location.

Caught completely off guard, the two U.S. foreign and domestic intelligence agencies, the CIA and FBI, had missed clues, failed to connect the dots, and didn't share intel with each other on the terrorist training camps overseas and the young male Saudi citizens learning how to fly planes without any interest in landing them. The United States was on the inexorable path to war against the terrorist mastermind, Osama bin Laden, and his al-Qaeda terror group. With President George W. Bush shutting down all commercial flights across the U.S. for two days to prevent further hijackings, a slew of bomb scares were called in, soon to be followed by envelopes of anthrax arriving at various news organizations in New York and Florida, among other states.

Within a week of the 9/11 terrorist attacks, in which the jets' fuel and air speed were turned into missiles, a more sinister, unnerving agent of terror was sent in nothing bigger than an envelope by U.S. Postal Services. The white powder of weapons-grade anthrax posed a different psychological tactic in warfare. Once some of the anthrax packages were opened, others were intercepted at various media companies, government agencies, and at the offices of a pair of politicians in then–Senate Majority Leader Tom Daschle (D-SD) and Senator Pat Leahy (D-VT)—the two senators who would oppose the passage of the U.S. Patriot Act. With the deaths of only five people and the infection of seventeen others, anthrax initially worked great at instilling terror but failed to be an effective airborne powder that could actually kill and maim hundreds, if not thousands of citizens.[98]

That dark reality never came to be.

As sudden as the terrorist attacks happened on the morning of 9/11, the CDC, for the first time in its existence after being founded

---

[98] "Vital Unresolved Anthrax Questions and ABC News" by Glenn Greenwald, Salon.com August 1, 2008.

in 1946 to combat malaria, was thrust into the military–intelligence industrial complex.

On October 24, then-CDC director Dr. Jeffrey Koplan was interviewed by news anchor Jim Lehrer on PBS to discuss the anthrax terrorist attacks. A minute after introductions, Koplan stumbles while talking out of both sides of his mouth in an unsure delivery at a time when the nation still needed reassuring.

"I think specimens are being taken and they're being examined and considered clinically in the hospital. But, again, we're trying to keep it very low sensitivity, or high sensitivity for people to come forth with any kind of illness particularly if they're postal."[99]

Anyone tuned into what the director of the CDC was trying to articulate would have had problems with that explanation. So what was it? Low sensitivity? Or high sensitivity? His next answer wasn't any better at restoring faith that a scientist could also be a good public speaker, a skillful messenger, and a seasoned politician. Dr. Koplan was none of the above.

"I characterize it as both relatively contained currently, but unpredictable—that's what we've seen, again in Florida with two cases there, one other person exposed, and located in one building; several instances of work sites namely related to the media in New York City; some spread and a very troubling spread in postal facilities—are still relatively circumscribed as a disease. I think a key feature of anthrax is it is not communicable person to person."[100]

Again, what was Dr. Koplan saying about the anthrax attacks? How were they paradoxically "contained" and "unpredictable" at the same time? It was hard to tell. Then he reassured viewers with this winner: "Some spread and a very troubling spread in postal facilities ..."

---

[99] "The Anthrax Threat: Dr. Jeffrey Koplan, Director of the CDC," PBS News Hour with Jim Lehrer, October 24, 2001.

[100] Ibid.

Back in 2001, the Internet and Amazon Prime hadn't replaced the utility of snail-mail quite yet. Little matter. With the pressure on the U.S. government to take the war to the terrorists and hunt Osama bin Laden in Afghanistan and to while quell the fears about the anthrax attacks, HHS's Director Tommy Thompson and President Bush must have rolled their eyes and shook their heads at what came out of the mouth of the CDC director.

Dr. Jeffrey Koplan could not lead the CDC in the new age of bio-terrorism. On February 12, 2002, Koplan resigned from the CDC as the health agency's thirteenth director.[101] With the search for a new director having begun, four interim co-directors were appointed to hold down the fort until a new director would be selected.

One of those four interim co-chiefs was Dr. Julie Louise Gerberding, an expert epidemiologist who led the CDC's response to the anthrax attacks in the wake of 9/11. Unlike Dr. Koplan, the slender, well-dressed, Glamour-elegant, forty-six-year-old scientist knew how to deal with the press, answer questions in a clear, articulate manner, and never showed strain or broke a sweat under the klieg lights of the media. With a shock of gray hair sprouting from the top of her fore-head giving her the skunk-like look of Looney Tunes cartoon char-acter Pepé le Pew, Dr. Julie Gerberding nonetheless had everything required to lead the CDC in a new direction in a new era of domestic and global threats from infectious diseases to manmade pestilence.

The *Lancet* Infectious Diseases wrote an editorial on Julie Gerberding in its "The Leading Edge" column, "A Time of Change at the CDC":

With infectious diseases perceived as a national security issue, something that was not the case 10 years ago, the time seems right for change at the CDC. So why was Gerberding chosen?

---

[101] "CDC Chief Jeffrey Koplon Resigns" by Erin McClam, Associated Press, February 2, 2002.

Unlike some of the previous 13 CDC directors, Gerberding's experience does not lie in the public-health system but in academic medicine and direct patient care. She worked as an infectious-disease specialist and epidemiologist for more than a decade with a career-long interest in prevention. Indeed, she is the first director with infectious disease subspecialty training and board certification. Her ability as a highly articulate and decisive spokeswoman who is calm and unruffled in the face of criticism was seen during the anthrax attacks, while representing the CDC to congress and the public.[102]

Born and raised in South Dakota, Julie Gerberding trained in internal medicine, infectious diseases, and clinical pharmacology at San Francisco General Hospital and the University of California, San Francisco. She would earn her master's degree in health at the University of California, Berkeley. After spending most of the 1990s as director of the Epidemiology and Prevention Interventions Center at San Francisco General, she joined the CDC in 1998, first working on guidelines for HIV infections with healthcare workers, then branching out to anthrax and bioterrorism.[103]

As the first woman director in the CDC's fifty-six-year history, Julie Gerberding inherited a "sea of troubles." By summer 2002, the U.S.-led invasion of Afghanistan had failed to kill or capture Osama bin Laden and other heads of the al-Qaeda terrorist network. A second front on war was developing in Iraq as intelligence sources indicated that Saddam Hussein was manufacturing weapons of mass destruction and bioweapons, including anthrax. Then add to that potent cocktail the avian bird flu scare, West Nile virus, childhood obesity epidemic,

---

[102] "A Time of Change at the CDC," Editorial in The Lancet Infectious Diseases, Vol. 2, August 2002.

[103] "Julie Gerberding Names Director of CDC" by Robert Ross, CIDRAP News, July 3, 2002.

autism epidemic, and parents weighing whether or not to vaccinate
their children . . . Dr. Gerberding had her hands full at the helm of the
agency. But if anyone could run the CDC and take it in a new direction while dealing with the media and general public, it was the girl
from South Dakota with German roots.

Before she was anointed director, a couple of behind the scenes
projects were already set in motion and gaining speed. First, the
Danish team began to finalize the paper "A Population-Based Study
of Measles, Mumps, and Rubella Vaccination and Autism" and submit
it to the prestigious *New England Journal of Medicine* (NEJM), to provide "strong evidence" that MMR vaccine doesn't cause autism. Bob
Wright's NAAR/Autism Speaks awarded $80,300 to Poul Thorsen at
Aarhus University to study the "Risk Factors for Neurodevelopmental
Disorders: MMR Vaccine & Childhood Autism."[104] That study would
sail through to publication in NEJM on November 7, 2002.

The second project, with the two thimerosal studies from Verstraeten
et al. and Madsen et al., had long roads still to travel. In the former study,
the CDC team continued to filter and flatten the data over and again
until the numbers would tip in their favor, showing no causation. The latter hit some turbulence, being turned down twice by *Lancet* and *JAMA*.
As these rejections cropped up in 2002, Julie Gerberding observed what
would happen next.

By year's end, it took NCBDDD director Jose Cordero's persuasive letter to strong-arm a third but less prestigious journal, *Pediatrics*,
to finally publish the "little paper," as Dr. Kreesten Madsen called
the study he led as principal investigator. Julie Gerberding let Diana
Schendel and her boss, Coleen Boyle, make sure the study would
get published, which included omitting the 2001 data that would
have distorted the final message—and the true results—of a likely link
between thimerosal and autism.

---

[104] Autism Speaks, 2002 Research Awards (NAAR), Pilot Study Grants to Poul
Thorsen.

Derived from the German personal name Gerbert, Julie Gerberding's surname translates to two words: "spear" and "bright."[105] The "Bright-Spear" was not going to get her hands soiled or bloodied. She would use other people to do the dirty work and employ foreign data to obtain favorable results outside the normal purview of the agency in order to keep any scientific blowback or controversy from touching her.

Julie Gerberding entrusted the completion of the Madsen thimerosal study to the hands of Drs. Coleen Boyle and Diana Schendel. In Boyle, the new director had the can't-find-a-link of causation between the plane flight paths of Agent Orange Operation Ranch Hand and the Vietnam veterans who got sick or ill with cancers on the ground. In Schendel, she had a scientist and epidemiologist who had gone through backtesting of data before in the Woburn Superfund site a dozen years before. Diana Schendel was only half way—ten more years—to getting her federal government pension. So she must have been a lieutenant Gerberding could lean on, like a soldier, at crunch time; an employee who would follow orders and not question them; a scientist who could think on the fly and solve problems with little oversight.

As the two major thimerosal studies got under way, Julie Gerberding thought she could set her sights on overhauling the moribund agency and transform it into managing the array of threats that it and the U.S. public would face in the coming years. Beyond the re-engineering of the agency for the twenty-first century, the director grasped that the CDC had to become better at messaging, staying ahead of stories, and spinning negative press into a positive sound bite.

The first such challenge came in late September. Stories broke in the news of how germs, bacteria, even anthrax had been shipped to Iraq, the country the second Bush president was about to go to war with for a second time since the original attack in the 1980s. Now

---

[105] http://www.ancestry.com/name-origin?surname=gerberding

the 2001 anthrax attacks and scare had returned like a boomerang one year after first emerging. Since this was an old problem with a different agency director two decades before she earned the right to be the CDC chief, Julie Gerberding was not about to let her corporate image and good name be tarnished in anyway. She appointed Tom Skinner, the CDC's media relations guru, to address the press and public on the hot issue.

"We ship over 300 agents to several dozen countries every year," said CDC spokesman Thomas Skinner. "It's important for the CDC to cooperate with international health authorities on research that . . . saves lives. At the same time it's equally important to us to work with the U.S. Commerce Department to see that these organisms don't fall into the wrong hands."[106]

The Commerce Department released a list of countries that were on the black list of international trade for germs, including Iran, Syria, Libya, Sudan, North Korea and Cuba. But during the 1980s, Iraq was an ally and so not on that do-not-send list.[107]

When that storm ended, a new one would emerge after the invasion of Iraq on March 9, 2003. Within months of entering the new theater for the War on Terror, an opportunistic pathogen in drug-resistant *Acinetobacter* began to emerge in field hospitals and medical tents in Iraq. The *Acinetobacter* infections in wounded soldiers began to spread around the country to other military healthcare facilities.[108]

Once extremely rare in the United States during the 1980s and 1990s, the superbug soon flourished. "As many as 40 percent of soldiers returning from the NATO mission in Afghanistan carry the

---

[106] "U.S. Like Sent Iraq Toxic Bugs," by Mike Toner, Atlanta-Journal Constitution, October 2, 2002.

[107] Ibid.

[108] "The Acinetobacter Threat," Bryant Furlow at EPI News, June 11, 2010.

bacteria, and it's commonly spread in field hospitals, resulting in pneumonia."[109]

What angered many people, including war veterans, was the CDC, in concert with the Pentagon, kept the superbug outbreak silent. Director Gerberding chose not to speak to the public about the dangers of the antibiotic bacteria, hold a presser, or even get ahead of the story. Perhaps the war in Iraq was enough bad news for Americans to stomach on a daily basis. Yet the superbug wouldn't stay in the battlefields for long. The pathogen hitched a ride with the returning soldiers and contractors, who would receive ongoing treatment, surgery, and physical therapy across the United States in doctors' offices, hospitals, emergency rooms, medical centers, nursing homes, schools, colleges, universities, and businesses, and pass the lethal germs along, as if people were trapped on board a flu-ridden cruise ship.

Not publicly sharing the bad news or reaching out to healthcare physicians, nurses and specialists across the country, the once rare disease had spread into the greater population, like Air Force planes from Operation Ranch Hand had been dispersing Agent Orange defoliant on the general public.

In each challenge or instance, Dr. Julie Gerberding knew when to take control of the communication for the CDC, when to pass it on—and distance herself by doing so—and when to withhold the information altogether. Whether by design or pressure from the White House or Joint Chiefs of Staff to go public with the deadly bug, Julie Gerberding, however unwittingly, had put the health of millions of Americans at risk and in the line of fire from the war zone of Iraq.

Early on in her post as new CDC chief, valuable insights enabled Gerberding to keep the Danish studies with Coleen Boyle, Diana Schendel, and the visiting scientist Poul Thorsen. In the budding relationship between Poul and Diana, no matter how hard the lovers tried to tone down their affection for one another, Julie Gerberding read

---

[109] "Three Canadian Soldiers Sick with Superbug" UPI, August 20, 2009.

their body language, tuned into the inflections of their voices, and saw the twinkle in their eyes, which were a direct pathway to their souls. Instead of either supporting or denouncing the courtship, Julie Gerberding needed the doctors' romance to flourish.

Doing so would create a buffer between them and her director's office in case a few years down the road blowback came from the Danish studies. Fall guys and scapegoats were always good insurance to have; foreign lackeys were the premium of those types of policies.

If the shit hit the fan with Poul Thorsen or his research group NANEA in Denmark, Gerberding figured all she had to do was turn the fan on high and step away from the mess, leaving him hanging out to dry.

# 11

# NANEA, NO PANACEA

Poul Thorsen and Diana Schendel were more than a couple of research scientists sharing the sheets, the sand at the coastal city of Aarhus during the summers in Denmark, and time together professionally in the lab or office, whether in Atlanta or Aarhus. They collaborated on many studies across a broad range of ailments, diseases, and disorders. The range of the studies became the basis for the research units within the Aarhus University research group North Atlantic Neuro-Epidemiology Alliances, or NANEA.

Before Dr. Julie Gerberding became director of the CDC, Dr. Poul Thorsen was thoroughly entrenched in the agency. He was more than a foreign visiting scientist. He had fully immersed his career and future in Atlanta, Georgia, earning his own U.S. federal government email address and becoming the principal investigator for a study funded by the CDC's new division of National Center of Birth Defects and Developmental Disabilities in the Developmental Disabilities Branch.

The study, "Identification of Biological/Biochemical Marker(s) for Preterm Delivery," by Dr. Poul Thorsen with Diana Schendel et al., was published in Blackwell Science, Ltd., Pediatric and Perinatal Epidemiology. Just like many of the future studies Thorsen's NANEA would work on, the U.S. would fund the research, while Thorsen leveraged the Danish Health Registries—specifically the regional Odense Cohort Study of 2,927 pregnant women in Denmark's third largest city.

The study was aimed at trying to identify biomarkers of certain women with risk of preterm delivery before thirty-seven weeks in gestation. "Knowledge gained from the proposed studies will be implemented in a third, clinical intervention study against PTD. The first phase of the clinical intervention study will be to establish a risk-assessment model based on the 'best' combination of biological/biochemical measures and other factors associated with PATG in order to identify pregnant women at very high risk of PTD,"[110] or preterm delivery.

Studies like this, researched with Diana Schendel, backed by the deep pockets of the CDC, and planned with more phases of research to come, gave Poul Thorsen clout inside and outside of the agency, in the United States and back home in Denmark and other European countries. It also gave him confidence to raise grant money outside of the CDC and gave him the impetus that he would soon no longer need the services of politically connected partner Ib Terp who, by 2004, eyed becoming mayor of the town of Brøndby as he had been connected to the city council since the late 1970s. Sure, Thorsen would still raise grant money from time to time from the Danish Medical Research Council, but they would be minor partners on the pot of gold that he would bring home with the Centers for Disease Control's desperate need to disprove theories, links, and facts about vaccine safety.

But in going it alone and leading his NANEA research group by himself without the supervision of Ib Terp or having a real business partner who would provide a back-office mooring and a sounding

---

[110] "Identification of Biological/Biochemical Marker(s) for Preterm Delivery," Dr. Poul Thorsen et al., Blackwell Science, Ltd., Paediatric and Perinatal Epidemiology, 2001 (Suppl. 2), 90-103.

board to generate revenue for new ideas, Poul Thorsen broke the first rule of steel tycoon Andrew Carnegie.

Napoleon Hill, a journalist who interviewed Carnegie toward the end of his life, discovered the one principle the steel magnet and philanthropist, and the richest man in the world at the time, would "credit all his riches," fame, and fortune to. It's a principle that, more than a hundred years later in the wealth of Silicon Valley, resonates today.

Hill defines the principle as, "Coordination of knowledge and effort, in a spirit of harmony, between two or more people, for the attainment of a definite purpose."

In other words, it means surrounding yourself with talented people who share your vision, because the alignment of several smart and creative minds is exponentially more powerful than just one.[111]

Without surrounding himself with a true business partner, Poul Thorsen would never be able to realize his dream of building a university research group into a leading powerhouse company in the field of datamining and epidemiology. He would have no one to reign him in, question his motives, stand up to him or challenge him when he did something wrong, stepped out of line, failed to execute a strategy, or worse. Poul Thorsen didn't surround himself at NANEA with talented people and sharp minds—quite the opposite. He hired a bunch of "yes" people, interns, low-wage managers, and paid consultants; the sharp analytical minds, such as Kreesten Meldgaard Madsen, Morgens Vestergaard, and Ulrik Kesmodel, were paid by Aarhus University and were even based there and not in NANEA's on-campus office. Eventually the office would move off-campus into a beautiful red-brick house up the hill from both the center of town and the Aarhus

---

[111] "The practice legendary tycoon Andrew Carnegie credits for his riches can be used by anyone," by Kathleen Elkins, Business Insider, June 26, 2015.

University School of Medicine, where Thorsen originally earned his masters of science, "master candi," the equivalent of a medical doctor degree in the United States with an internship to follow. Poul Thorsen was an average scientist, an unknown doctor in a country of thousands of topflight research doctors, physicians, PhDs, and other specialists. He wouldn't have stood out, not as a scientist in his early forties against older, smarter, more experienced, and award-winning researchers with hundreds of published studies in their belt with lifetimes of achievement.

With NANEA moving off-campus and Thorsen's "me-style" flamboyance with a salesman delivery, he raised eyebrows, ruffled the feathers of his peers, and made his elder statesmen jealous and envious, creating resentment amongst the ranks. But it cemented Poul Thorsen's rising stature as some kind of scientific dealmaker. His work ultimately was based on the money he brought to Aarhus University, not on his brief tenure or his less than stellar research, research that seemed impressive in name, title, and subject matter but not in the science itself. From my research, Poul Thorsen was not a patent holder. His name didn't conjure up any breakthrough science, nor did it crown him with any awards or accolades.

For most of his life, Poul Thorsen was an average scientist. Yet in surrounding himself with "yes" people—the cheap, young, inexperienced folks at NANEA—his lightweight knowledge of science wouldn't be enough to bail him out of tight jams.

# I 2

# THE DANE AND THE DICTATOR

"Borderlands of the Danes" refers to "a political unit created during the sixth through ninth centuries,"[112] or what is known as the Viking Age of Scandinavia.

Those endearing Vikings, before they set out to map Western Europe by the sea via raids, trading voyages, and other sea-treks beyond Denmark's continental shelf, "marked" the borders of the Jutland peninsula to the south along the trading center of Hedeby, near the German border. The strands, coastlines, and littoral bends in bays and coves were natural borders, as were many of the islands that makeup Denmark today, along with parts of southern Norway and Sweden.

Dr. Julie Louis Gerberding might not have been an expert on Norse history, nor have the lineage of a Viking queen, but she knew how to sail her own ship, beach it, and then draw up her own boundaries. In less than five years, she went from working as an epidemiologist at the CDC on HIV and then bioterrorism to running the entire agency.

---

[112] http://www.everyculture.com/Cr-Ga/Denmark.html – Section:'Orientation' Subsection:'Identification.'

She was fortunate that 9/11 happened during her career, because it was out of that tragic event and ensuing anthrax attacks that President George W. Bush and Tommy Thompson, the director of HHS, noticed her. And so her profile rose within the agency during the dark autumn after the al-Qaeda attacks.

It was the plotting within the Bush Administration to take the War on Terror outside the land that al-Qaeda operated that separated Gerberding from other candidates to run the CDC in a new era of asymmetrical warfare and other threats.

Contrary to published reports that President Bush created the Islamic State of Iraq and al-Sham (ISIS)—he did not—it was the Jordanian terrorist Abu Musab al-Zarqawi who rose through the ranks of al-Qaeda to become the founder of ISIS. First trained by Osama bin Laden in Afghanistan and then funded by him to open and manage terrorist training camps after the U.S. invasion of Afghanistan, by spring 2002 al-Zarqawi was training locals and foreign fighters for jihad in northern Iraq.[113]

For Julie Gerberding stepping into the director's chair, she knew two things. One, the team of CDC PhD scientists—Drs. Coleen Boyle, Bill Thompson, Frank DeStefano, Bob Chen, Diana Schendel, Marshalyn Yeargin-Allsopp, and others—were what the U.S. Navy would call, in its unique blue jargon, "puke lifers," since they would work for the agency until retirement and pension collection. Dr. Gerberding wanted no part of being at the agency that long. Second, she had been given carte blanche by the Bush Administration to overhaul an analog agency to meet the challenges of the Digital Age.

Like the Vikings of "Den-mark," Julie Gerberding went ahead to mark her boundaries, redistricting some business units within the CDC, repurposing others, as if they were neighborhoods in a small town. She rubbed and ruffled peers, scientists, and staff with the

---

[113] http://www.historycommons.org/context.jsp?item=a1102noattackagain

changes she made because she had the full support of President Bush and Tommy Thompson—and knew it.

When the librarian-looking Coleen Boyle needed the help of NCBDDD Director Jose Cordero—to write the persuasive letter to journal *Pediatrics* to get them to both fast-track and publish the Danish Thimerosal Study—Gerberding didn't want her name on any of those emails. Of course, the director backed the position of the agency to erase any links between thimerosal and rising autism rates, as they had done with the MMR Studies conducted by Tom Verstraeten and Kreesten Madsen, with the latter being published in the *New England Journal of Medicine* on November 7, 2002. Julie just didn't want her name on part of any future email chain that might be exposed years later under the Freedom of Information Act.

Two days before Thanksgiving 2002, Boyle wrote an email to Jose Cordero, with the subject: "Autism Thimerosal Paper – Cover Letter."

"I will prepare the letter for Jose's signature—but won't get to it until next week. I would suggest that it accompany the submission as support of the importance of the work. I can fedex [*sic*] it so it arrives late next week.

"Jose: We need to discuss. Thx. Coleen Boyle, PhD."[114]

Julie Gerberding would let her minions do her bidding. And as for Poul Thorsen and the Danish Team, as long as they were paid to backtest historical data from the Danish Health Registries on subjects of the CDC's choosing and shown how to slant those studies, then she was all in for going the safe route. Let foreigners conduct the studies overseas with their data, have CDC scientists like Diana Schendel and Coleen Boyle oversee the results of those studies prior to submitting them to journals to be so-called "peer-reviewed" and published.

By the time 2003 came around and the U.S. invaded Iraq for a second time in as many decades, pressure mounted from the parents of

---

[114] Email Nov. 26, 2002: From CDC Coleen Boyle to NCBDDD Jose Cordero, "Autism Thimerosal Paper – Cover Letter."

the growing autism community to get answers on what was happening to their children and the ballooning vaccine bubble. It was in that vein that Julie Gerberding familiarized herself with the documents that the CDC shared with Poul Thorsen and NANEA.

Knowing that the Madsen thimerosal study wouldn't be published for months in *Pediatrics*—which meant deep into the new year even with Jose Cordero's forceful letter—and that Congress circled the U.S. vaccine program looking for answers to the autism epidemic, Julie Gerberding couldn't take the chance that the study wouldn't be published. So she looked for backup plans that included more studies to be conducted in Denmark. Rummaging through the history prior to her being director of the CDC, Gerberding picked up a nine-page letter from the CDC to a man named Ib Terp at the Danish Medical Research Council. The sender of the letter was Lisa T. Garbarino, grant management specialist at the agency. Copying Diana Schendel on the letter, it began:

"Dear Mr. Terp:

"Enclosed is your cooperative agreement award under Program Announcement #00013 'Determination of the Relationship Between Infection in Pregnancy and Cerebal [*sic*] Palsy.'"[115]

Like Dr. Diane Simpson who couldn't spell the word "thimerosal" correctly for a month, a major typo appeared in the opening sentence from the CDC. Not that the Danes cared about the lack of a spell check on the Word document as long as the CDC money was sent to them, but it was embarrassing for even the erstwhile supervisor of NANEA to bear.

To secure the Danish scientists full cooperation going forward, Julie Gerberding knew she had to increase the funds to them—a lot more than several million over a number of years—going beyond the usual process of writing a grant and waiting for the money to come

---

[115] "Dec 23 1999: Cerebal [*sic*] Palsy Letter from U.S. CDC to Ib Terp, DK," by Ulla Danielsen, December 23, 2014.

after green lighting a new study. She knew Diana Schendel's lover would be game. That "continuation" or second cooperative agreement between the CDC and NANEA, by way of Ib Terp's Danish Research Council, was going to be big dollars-wise: Eight-plus million dollars in aggregate going back to the start of 2000 and the first cooperative agreement, and deep into the second half of the decade. With Thorsen using the CDC as his golden sponsor, it allowed him, it motivated him, it got him juiced to go out and find and secure more grant money both in the States and in Denmark, across the North Sea in the United Kingdom and across the European Union.

The CDC legitimized Poul Thorsen as a research scientist. In doing so, it fed the Dane, who was an attention grabber, a capitalist in a conservative, socialist society. Thorsen's quest for money and fame, or at least name recognition, made him an outlier in Danish society.

Poul Thorsen's brainchild, NANEA, looked great, even stellar, to the outside world—at least on paper. On the NANEA website in 2002, which was hosted and paid for by Aarhus University, it boasted five different research units, each with a team leader. They included Alcohol, Autism, Cerebral Palsy, Preterm Delivery, and Special Projects. There were twenty-four employees at the time, plus Ib Terp serving in the role of supervisor, even though he had zero interaction with the rest of the staff and employees as he was based in Copenhagen, which by train is more than three hours away from Aarhus.[116]

What the CDC didn't know and Diana Schendel did, who spent several summers there, along with Drs. Diane Simpson, Paul Stehr-Green, and Marshalyn Yeargin-Allsopp, was that Thorsen was able to show them and any other visitors from the CDC that NAENA was fully operational. But that was within Aarhus University campus. And

---

[116] http://web.archive.org/web/20021215062608/http:/www.nanea.dk/team/team_aarhus.html

without either the CDC or Aarhus University asking Poul Thorsen for annual accounting statements, the reality was quite different than the perception of how greatly knitted, built, and fed NANEA really was.

In interviewing the team leader for the autism research unit in Kreesten Meldgaard Madsen—the first time any journalist inside or out of Denmark spoke to him about his years working with Thorsen and NANEA—at the end of June 2015, he said that "Poul Thorsen had all this money from the CDC, yet he starved his research group NANEA. I was paid by Aarhus University, just like other quality scientists. At NANEA, he hired mid level managers and lots of interns. Poul Thorsen starved NANEA," he repeated during the thirty-minute interview.

But Thorsen's house of cards was out of sight in Denmark. Add Ib Terp's name and solid reputation with the Danish Research Council and the century-old Aarhus University, and he felt there was no way for the CDC or anyone else to question the validity of his research, NANEA's lofty goals, and, in the end, what he did with the money or how he spent it. Still in 2003, he had to go secure the second phase of the international cooperative agreement.

In the U.S., there was trouble brewing for the CDC as Congress Research Service produced a report on May 12, 2003, titled, "Mercury in Products and Waste: Legislative and Regulatory Activities to Control Mercury."

Mercury, such as thimerosal, would be back in the headlines and national consciousness that summer and fall. There was no getting around it. And in the fourteen-page abstract, the news wasn't good concerning how long the CDC, FDA, and vaccine manufacturers could continue to pull the wool over the eyes of the American people . . . and if failing to do that, what it would take to fool, mask, or condition the mainstream press to be on the side of Goliath over David. The summary of the study read, "Mercury is a highly volatile, naturally-occurring element. It is a potent neurotoxin that can cause brain, lung, and kidney damage. Mercury also has properties that make it useful in a variety of household, medical, and industrial products and processes. It is a component in such products as thermometers, fluorescent [sic] lamps, electrical switches, dental fillings, and batteries."[117]

The abstract rambled on for several pages on organic versus inorganic, vapor and dental work to pollution and industrial waste. Finally it arrived at vaccines and thimerosal. On page CRS-9, they wrote:

> There has been legislative activity in both the 107th and 108th Congress related to the use of mercury in childhood vaccines, particularly the presence of the mercury-containing preservative thimerosal. A provision added to the Homeland Security Act (P.L. 107-296), which revised the Public Health Service Act (42 U.S.C. 300), was interpreted as protecting vaccine manufacturers from potential financial liability related to the use of thimerosal. The preservative is added to formulations for influenza, diphtheria-tetanus, tetanus, hepatitis B, and rabies. Opponents of the provision argued that it would effectively end lawsuits for injuries caused to children after multiple mercury exposures from thimerosal in infant vaccines. On January 10, 2003, Senators Olympia Snowe, Susan Collins, and Lincoln Chafee announced an agreement with Senate leadership to address concerns that arose from the addition of the vaccine-related language. The language in P.L. 107-296 was subsequently removed in the Consolidated Appropriations Resolution for 2003 (P.L. 108-7).[118]

On March 19, 2003, Representative Dan Burton introduced the National Vaccine Injury Compensation Program Improvement Act of 2003 (H.R. 1349). The bill would amend the Public Health

---

[117] "Mercury Products and Waste: Legislative and Regulatory Activities to Control Mercury," Linda G. Luther, Environmental Policy Analyst, Resources, Science, and Industry Division. May 12, 2003, pg. 2 (provided by Wikileaks.org).

[118] Ibid, CRS-9.

Service Act (42 U.S.C. 300) with respect to the National Vaccine Injury Compensation Program (VICP), by extending the statute of limitations on filing claims for vaccine-related injuries, and increasing the base amount of funding available to those injured. While the bill does not refer to concerns about thimerosal specifically, Representative Burton has discussed, in hearings and publications, the connection between the exposure to the mercury- containing preservative and neurological developmental disorders of autism, and speech and language delays.[119]

The Conclusion of the report, its last sentences, drove home what need to be done across the board by all federal agencies.

"Both federal and state authorities have taken action to control the introduction of mercury into the environment that originates from the use of mercury in products and manufacturing processes. The current trend, in many federal and state legislative actions, is to reduce mercury releases by eliminating it altogether, either from its use in manufacturing processes or as an added component to products. Many states have passed such legislation; few federal initiatives have been enacted into law."[120]

The line to "eliminate mercury altogether" took place across the board in the United States and would accelerate under the Obama Administration to reduce the dependence on coal and the number of coal-fired power plants significantly. It happened with the dentists of America, it happened in thermometers, and it happened in other chemical processes.

But the one place mercury was still alive and well—since it was never banned from vaccines, merely reduced on an honor system—were in vaccines meant for pregnant women, unborn fetuses, and newborn babies.

---

[119] Ibid, CRS-9-10.
[120] Ibid, CRS-11.

## I 3

# SAFETY IN NUMBERS

This final recommendation of the Committee Report is most troubling because it highlights an ongoing double standard applied by the Human Resources Subcommittee regarding the work of scientists, both inside and outside of government. The implications of this double standard are clear: If you're a scientist who agrees with the political conclusions of the Human Resources Subcommittee Chairman, your views will be put forth as gospel, and no one has a right to question them. On the other hand, if you're a scientist who disagrees with the Chairman's political conclusions, you'll either be lucky enough to be ignored, or you'll face the unfortunate prospects of having your views attacked and your integrity questioned before a publicly held Congressional hearing.

We are simply tired of seeing Administration officials constantly dragged through the Human Resources Subcommittee wringer under the banner of science over politics, when the Subcommittee is the one so clearly guilty of playing politics itself.

Veterans deserve much better than what this report seeks to offer.[121]

This text could have easily been written in the twenty-first century by the senators and congressmen who met with CDC, FDA, NIH, and IOM officials, and parents of spectrum children, trying to get to the bottom of the vaccine safety issue. But instead of being part of Senator Dan Burton's (R-IN from 1983-2013) March 2003 hearings or the February 2004 IOM hearings on "Vaccines and Autism," the passage was written by the six dissenting senators in 1990 who went on the record to complain about the lack of findings and connections between dioxin of Agent Orange and the ill health and rare, acute cancers of too many U.S. Vietnam War veterans and the lack of accountability in the Centers for Disease Control, which facilitated the epidemiological studies.

The six senators were:

> Richard K. Armey
> Frank Horton
> Howard C. Nielson
> J. Dennis Hasert
> Jon L. Kyl
> Chuck Douglas[122]

Surprising in retrospect, the same Senator "Dick" Armey, who stood up for the abused and injured and forgotten Vietnam veterans, decided in 2002 to go over to the dark side and protect the industrial pharmacologist complex rather than the little guys—Senator Armey stood up against the poisoning of U.S. Army troops, yet a dozen years later didn't stand up for the little, little guys—as in babies, infants, toddlers, and children.

---

[121] "The Agent Orange Coverup: A Case of Flawed Science and Political Manipulation, the Twelfth Report by the Committee on Government Operations." together with Dissenting Views, Pg. 42-43 (8-9-1990) 101ˢᵗ Congress.

[122] Ibid, pg. 43

Under the storm of the growing autism–thimerosal divide at the turn of the millennium, where the autism incidence rates for newborns were rising each year as if it was a compounded double digit growth investment, Senator Richard Armey (R-TX), wrote a rider into his Homeland Security Act of 2002 after the 475-page bill was done.

The two paragraphs on pages 472 and 473 of the Act (H.R. 5005), born out of a response to the 9/11 terrorist attacks, read:

*"Sec. 1714. Clarification of Definition of Manufacturer.* Section 2133(3) of the Public Health Service Act (42 U.S.C. 300aa–33(3)) is amended—

"(1) in the first sentence, by striking "under its label any vaccine set forth in the Vaccine Injury Table" and inserting "any vaccine set forth in the Vaccine Injury table, including any component or ingredient of any such vaccine"; and

"(2) in the second sentence, by inserting "including any component or ingredient of any such vaccine" before the period."[123]

*"Sec. 1715. Clarification of Definition of Vaccine-Related Injury of Death*

Section 2133(5) of the Public Health Service Act (42 U.S.C. 300aa–33(5)) . . .

"is amended by adding at the end the following: "For purposes of the preceding sentence, an adulterant or contaminant shall not include any component or ingredient listed in a vaccine's product license application or product label."

*"Sec. 1716. Clarification of Definition of Vaccine.* Section 2133 of the Public Health Service Act (42 U.S.C. 300aa–33) is amended by adding at the end the following:

The term "vaccine" means any preparation or suspension, including but not limited to a preparation or suspension containing an attenuated or inactive microorganism or subunit thereof

---

[123] Homeland Security Act of 2002 (H.R. 5005), November 25, 2002, pgs. 472-73.

or toxin, developed or administered to produce or enhance the body's immune response to a disease or diseases and includes all components and ingredients listed in the  vaccines's product license application and product label.[124]

The rider was written in the night, as in the "night rider," and the bill was voted in the House on Monday, November 25, 2002— the very short holiday week. It was the week of America's biggest, non-religious, non-denominational holiday of Thanksgiving. Just as reporters and journalists were reviewing what George W. Bush had signed into law, Coleen Boyle wrote the email to Jose Cordero on creating the letter he would sign and send to *Pediatrics*, accompanying the Danish thimerosal study.

After Thanksgiving break, Arianna Huffington reacted as follows to the protect-the-vaccine-manufacturers' rider:

"Everyone in D.C., it seems, is utterly baffled as to how an ugly little provision shielding pharmaceutical behemoth Eli Lilly from billions in lawsuits filed by the parents of autistic children made its way, in the 12th hour, into, of all things, the 475-page Homeland Security bill.

"'It's a mystery to us,' shrugged Eli Lilly spokesman Rob Smith.

"It's a mystery to us, too, echoed spokesmen for the White House, the Department of Health and Human Services, and physician-turned-senator-turned-drug-company-shill Bill Frist, who had originally penned the Lilly-friendly provision for a different bill."[125]

Richard Armey's name was mentioned with other senators at the time, so who put in the rider remained a guarded secret until Dick Armey came out.

Online journal Tompaine.com offered a $10,000 reward to anyone identifying who inserted the rider into the bill. On National Public

---

[124] Ibid 473.

[125] "Expect no Patent Law revision in Eli Lilly's Washington," by Arianna Huffington, Dec. 4, 2002, http://islet.org/forum030/messages/27814.htm.

Radio (NPR) on December 19, 2002, Bill Moyers said, "Top of the list has to be Senator Frist. . . . Representative Armey has claimed credit (but) he's most likely just providing cover for somebody else who's sticking around after Armey leaves."[126]

CBS reported:

"I did it and I'm proud of it," says Armey, R-Texas. "It's a matter of national security," Armey says. "We need their vaccines if the country is attacked with germ weapons."

Rep. Dan Burton, R-Ind., isn't buying it. The grandfather of an autistic child, Burton says Armey slipped the provision in at the last minute, too late for debate. "And I said, 'Who told you to put it in?' He said, 'No, they asked me to do it at the White House.'"[127]

For new CDC Director Julie Gerberding, the "Lilly Rider," as it was referred to, signaled the next phase in shutting parents out of getting compensation for their vaccine-injured babies and children. She knew, however, there would be a fight ahead in Capitol Hill in 2003. Yet in the same breath, Gerberding saw to it that the CDC would push hard to get the Danish thimerosal study—Kreesten Madsen's baby—published.

In March 2003, Senator Dan Burton tried to override the Lilly Rider. In doing so, he met resistance both in the Senate and the White House, not to mention from the CDC and big pharma monolith.

By summer 2003, CDC Chief Julie Gerberding sat in a powerful position. The U.S. had invaded Iraq and begun a second front on the War of Terror. Since the anthrax attacks only claimed five lives—more people in the U.S. died that year in one hour[128] of car accidents in

---

[126] NOW with Bill Moyers, NPR, December 19, 2002.

[127] The Man Behind the Vaccine Mystery by Joel Roberts, December 12, 2002.

[128] http://www.cdc.gov/mmwr/preview/mmwrhtml/su6001a10.htm

the United States—the threat of weaponized anthrax was a doubtful proposition. A car bomb full of fertilizer was far more lethal than airborne anthrax spores. On the autism epidemic, she would wait patiently until the fall for the Danish thimerosal study to be published in peer-review process by the journal *Pediatrics*.

So when Dr. Gerberding was asked to speak at the eighth annual Richard J. Duma/NFID Press Conference and Symposium on Infectious Diseases, she accepted, joining a half dozen experts in their fields of epidemiology. But instead of focusing her talk on autism spectrum disorders, she chose to take the wake of 9/11 attacks with the topic on "21st Century Public Health: What is the New Normal."

While she focused on the "new normal" in the Age of Terrorism, Dr. Gerberding touched on old themes of bioterror, the potential weaponization of diseases, and how the rule of law was intended to protect the public, when in fact the new era empowered governments to spy on their citizens with little repercussion.

Dr. Boyle had experienced surviving the Senate gauntlet of the 1990 report on the failure of the CDC to find a link between the spraying of the dioxin aerosols during Operation Ranch Hand and the Vietnam veterans, getting promoted year after year while burying findings until one day she would take the director's chair after Jose Cordero in the new NCBDDD, a branch of CDC chartered in 2000 under the Clinton Administration that strictly focused on birth defects and developmental issues of newborn babies.

That mid summer day, Dr. Roger Glass upstaged the agency's first woman director when he took the podium one hour after Gerberding, and spoke on "Norovirus: An Emerging Viral Pathogen." With a background at the CDC in the Division of Viral and Rickettsia Diseases National Center for Infectious Diseases, he said:

> Diarrheal diseases remain among the most common afflictions of mankind. In developing countries, diarrhea remains the second most common cause of death among children, responsible

for more than 2 million deaths each year. In the US, it remains a common problem as well, with more than 70 million episodes, 500,000 hospitalizations and some 5,000 deaths occurring each year. Until recently, the etiology of a majority of these illnesses could not be determined; the recognized bacteria and parasites accounted for fewer than 20% of all outbreaks and hospitalizations.[129]

Again, the number of deaths, hospitalizations, and outbreaks blow away any year in-year out statistics on so-called measles outbreaks, with tens of people, sometimes hundreds of them, getting infected by the disease and fewer than a handful of deaths that mirrored the overhyped anthrax attacks, which in the end didn't make a very lethal biological weapon.

None of that made any difference to Julie Gerberding. What she learned in the first half of 2003 was what Dr. Coleen Boyle learned as a principal investigator in the Agent Orange debacle. Knowing Boyle survived a toothless Congress, Gerberding understood that the CDC was a Teflon monolith. Nothing could dent the agency or slow it down. That gave the director impetus to take risks within the CDC, overhaul sluggish parts of the agency, and take control of messaging without the fear of being fired when on the receiving end of political retribution or negative publicity.

Without being reckless or overconfident, Julie Gerberding knew 2003 was the year that the CDC would kill the thimerosal controversy with respect to vaccines while continuing to use Poul Thorsen's Danish team of scientists that they needed to produce whatever results the agency needed to produce. For Dr. Thorsen, 2003 was a pivotal year to renew or extend the cooperative agreement with the CDC. Although

---

[129] The 8th Richard J. Duma/NFID Annual Press Conference and Symposium on Infectious Diseases, "Norovirus: An Emerging Viral Pathogen," by Roger I. Glass, MD, at the National Press Club, Washington, DC, July 16, 2003.

she didn't want to sit at the negotiating table, she let it be known to Coleen Boyle and Diana Schendel that they needed to secure a deal but at a fair and equitable price, according to a source within the CDC.

On November 13, 2003, Tom Horne, MPH, deputy director at NCBDDD, wrote an email to Diana Schendel, who was in Denmark visiting Poul Thorsen and NANEA. It read:

> Diana, I hope all is well in Denmark (it must be a great relief to be there!) I need the Tech Review on the Danish application ASAP because I have to get signatures on the funding memo. Also, will human subjects tracking form change because of the application content? If not I can complete and obtain signoff. Thanks. Tom.[130]

The Tech Review was the next payment application for the cooperative agreement between the CDC and Poul Thorsen's NANEA. Busy at Aarhus University in Denmark, Diana Schendel replied three days later with a page-long email, writing:

"Tom, Here's the technical report. Plus I have attached two other files. The one called 'NANEA budget FY04' breaks out the budget by alcohol/CP/autism activities so you can see how it works out into separate piles."[131]

Schendel's "files" referred to research units within the NANEA research group. She went on to explain how the monies were allocated "equally" between the three units, with "CP" being cerebral palsy. She discussed increasing the international travel for the 2004 budget, "in order to pay for all costs (not expected to share with CDC, as has happened in past years).

"I have had long discussions with Poul on this trip about the budget—especially moving some of the lab costs into the future. I

---

[130] Email Nov. 13, 2003: From CDC Tom Horne to CDC Diana Schendel, "Application Tech Review."

[131] Ibid, Nov. 16, 2003.

think we will be able to get funds from the ELSASS Foundation to cover some of this in on future."[132]

Diana Schendel also mentioned the "weak dollar exchange rate doesn't help either."[133] She gave her itinerary to Horne, explaining she would be available on the phone Monday, travel back to the U.S. Tuesday, be in Washington, DC, Wednesday and Thursday, before flying back home to Atlanta on Friday.

When Tom Horne downloaded and opened the attachment in Schendel's email that Monday morning, he scanned the title: "Technical Reviewer Evaluation Report" Program Announcement: 0266, Epidemiological Studies of Reproductive and Developmental Outcomes—Denmark. Cooperative Agreement Number: UR3/CCU018305-05.[134]

It was labeled a "non-competing Continuation Report."

Poul Thorsen was in a no-bid, one-horse race to secure major funding from the CDC—again—as long as he played ball. On the report listed as "principal investigators" were Ib Terp and Poul Thorsen. But by the time the agreement would be signed in 2004, it would only contain Poul Thorsen's signature. With Terp moving into local politics the upcoming year, Poul Thorsen finally would be alone at the top, in charge of NANEA and in charge of invoicing for funds when certain milestones were reached. The supervision of the seasoned political animal Ib Terp would soon be gone: he left to become mayor of Brøndby.

The Tech Report application's brief overview read:

The application from the Danish Medical Research Council is for continuation of activities to investigate risk factors for adverse reproductive and developmental outcomes using the unique

---

[132] Ibid.

[133] Ibid.

[134] CDC "Technical Review Evaluation Report" to Danish Medical Research Council, November 17, 2003.

research sources in place in Denmark. The activities include studies of: 1) autism in relation to exposure of measles-mumps-rubella
(MMR) vaccine and potential biomarkers for autism measured on
newborn blood spots, taking other perinatal factors into account;
2) the relation between infection and the inflammatory response
of the mother and the fetus during pregnancy and the risk of cerebral palsy; and 3) the relation between level, pattern and timing
of prenatal fetal alcohol exposure and developmental outcome.
The application included descriptions of progress in each activity,
problems encountered and their solutions, objectives for the new
budget period, updates in administrative issues, an evaluation plan,
and a detailed budget and justification.[135]

The "unique research sources" was merely the Danish Health
Registries, which allowed Denmark, at the CDC's behest, to skew, manipulate, omit, cook, massage, and flatten the data until it read just right. Dr.
Diane Simpson had done her part to look for, interview, recruit, and
secure Denmark as the foreign taskmaster to deconstruct any passive or
causal links between autism and both MMR and thimerosal. More critical to securing the funding from the CDC was Diana Schendel's role in
writing the brief overview of the technical report. It was her professional
understanding of how the grant application would be reviewed and what
the key ingredients were to get it approved, and not Poul Thorsen, with
the visiting scientist's filling out that form that got the job done.

One week after Thanksgiving, the CDC emailed Poul Thorsen the
two-page "NANEA-CDC Cooperative Agreement, Budget: Year 3,
Feb 2004–Jan 2005."

The agreement's second to last paragraph on page two read, "We
will apply for the lack of funding outlined in the budget."[136]

---

[135]  Ibid.

[136]  "NANEA-CDC Cooperative Agreement, Budget: Year 3, Feb 2004–Jan
2005," December 6, 2003, page 2.

The last paragraph qualified that in the event of NANEA failing to get compensatory funding within six months that "we will change the study design according to the budget available, off [*sic*] course stop the data entry and cleaning process, not facilitate any international travel for project personnel, remove major technical support (mostly computer and software), not to request data from the Danish National Birth Cohort or from other Danish national registries for the lifestyle project, bit also remove the project from our projects' synergistic activities as not to handicap other projects, which is running in NANEA by the lack of funding in the Lifestyle project." Lifestyle referred to the alcohol studies.

Poul Thorsen wrote this last paragraph by himself, without the help of American Dr. Diana Schendel. The forging ahead of the studies, he knew, depended on money that he was confident to raise. With the CDC and Danish Medical Research Council at Aarhus University all in his corner, he would have little trouble securing additional funds needed to go forward. But the most telling line in his paragraph centered on the removal of the project from "our [NANEA] project's synergistic activities." That illusion, that power of perception Thorsen wrote into the agreement, would one day be proven a fallacy by a principal investigator on several of his key studies.

Unaware of future consequences for his actions—with Ib Terp out, the CDC money in, Diana Schendel in love with him, and CDC Director Julie Gerberding kept at a distance without asking serious questions about NANEA's work—Poul Thorsen felt he had finally made it. So did many at Aarhus University and within his research group NANEA.

On December 6, 2003, Poul Thorsen signed as the principal investigator for the cooperative agreement that would renew itself as long as Julie Gerberding was the CDC director. NANEA at the Department of Epidemiology and Social Medicine at Aarhus University was beginning to reach its apex as a research group that acted more like a Silicon Valley tech startup.

# I 4

# RISE OF THE MERCURY GODS

There are several metals that are natural to the human body. "In astronomy, defining a 'metal' is any element other than hydrogen or helium. Astronomers feel justified in grouping this diverse group of chemicals together because they only contribute 2% of the atomic matter in the universe."[137]

For macro elements the body is composed of calcium, phosphorous, magnesium, sodium, potassium, chlorine, and sulfur; on the micro scale iron, copper, manganese, iodine, zinc, selenium, fluorine, cobalt, molybdenum, and chromium populate our blood, bone, and flesh.[138] Nowhere on this empirical list of elements can one find the heavy earth metals of lead, mercury, cadmium, and arsenic—the elements among those blown out of the smoldering ruins of the 9/11 fires at Ground Zero. They also do not exist naturally; humans are not born with these metals. That can also be said about aluminum and mercury found in vaccines—they do not belong in our blood, sinew, and bone marrow.

---

[137] http://www.mendability.com/articles/our-brain-and-metals/
[138] Ibid.

The earth metals are not part of the evolution of the human species. And since heavy metals can be found in their purest forms when broken down, volatilized, or pulverized, they cannot be destroyed, vaporized or become soluble to be easily excreted by some process of the human body, such as urine, bowel movements, and perspiration through the skin pores. In fact, those metals, like drugs, can be tested for and found in human hair growth months after environmental insult as labs can do.

The protection of mercury-containing vaccines at all costs, as if they are "dolphin-safe" tuna, has been a disingenuous argument made by the CDC and FDA at bare minimum. Instead of joining the Scandinavian countries and Japan in banning thimerosal back in 1992, the US, through the Teflon CDC, has quadrupled down on the mercury-based preservative, like the agency had been guarding the health benefits of vitamins or nutrients. Today, many of the once TCV shots have been labeled to read "thimerosal-depleted."

What does that mean? It simply means that thimerosal is still used in the process of manufacturing vaccines but is strained or removed at the end of the process. So the reality that some vaccines are thimerosal-free is not quite true. Trace amounts can be found and can do harm to a subset of babies, children, and adults, as the documentary film of the same name, *Trace Amounts*, convincingly laid with overwhelming circumstantial evidence in 2015.

"Two forms of 'preservative-free vaccine packaged in single-dose presentations are available. One is manufactured without thimerosal (Fluzone, Sanofi-Aventis). In the other, thimerosal is removed at the end of the manufacturing process (Fluarix, GlaxoSmithKline). Almost all of the influenza vaccines administered to pregnant women in the 2005-2006 influenza season contained thimerosal at the preservative level.'[139]

---

[139] "Influenza Vaccination During Pregnancy: A Critical Assessment of the Recommendations of the Advisory Committee on Immunization Practices (ACIP)," by David M. Ayoub, MD, F. Ed Yazbak, MD, *Journal of American Physicians and Surgeons*, Vol. 11, No. 2, Summer 2006.

From the quadrupling down by the CDC on preserving thimerosal for the vaccine makers and serving them to fetuses and pregnant women via flu shot jabs that often don't work came this gem:

On May 28, 2004, the Advisory Committee on Immunization Practice (ACIP) of the Centers for Disease Control and Prevention (CDC) published its annual report on its current policy for prevention of influenza. The recommendation to vaccinate all pregnant women regardless of trimester was the most aggressive in a series of policy changes that began in 1995. Previously, influenza vaccine was advised only for women with preexisting medical conditions. The latest ACIP recommendation was promptly endorsed by the American College of Obstetricians and Gynecologists (ACOG) and the American Academy of Pediatrics (AAP).[140]

Thimerosal won again, despite the skyrocketing rates of autism spectrum disorders.

Senator Dick Armey's "Lilly Rider," which protected not defenseless babies, infants, and children but the vaccine manufacturers, wasn't even the last step in the federal government worshipping the mercury god thimerosal. The Danish studies were key to trying to cajole, convince, persuade, and bamboozle the general public and mainstream press that all vaccines were safe (they are not), that they had all been tested for safety (not one clinical trial on vaccinated and unvaccinated babies has ever been performed), and that there is no limit to the number of vaccines babies can receive on a single visit or over the course of their lives (again, this is patently false).

Had any of these statements been true, then the compensation of vaccine-injured babies, children, and people would never have been chartered in the National Vaccine Injury Compensation Program

---

[140] Ibid.

(NVCIP) Act of 1986 or formed with special masters running "Vaccine Court," which as of March 2014 has paid out north of $2.8 billion in damages.[141]

That excludes, with the stroke of a pen based on the cooked Danish Studies, the 5,400-plus thimerosal-injured cases dismissed by the Vaccine Court Omnibus—one which included my autistic son, born in 2000, who was damaged by thimerosal.

"As with over 5,400 other petitions, Dayton's [case] was dismissed in October 2011. She found this out by talking with a few advocates who were monitoring the OAP (Omnibus Autism Proceedings) and the subsequent dismissals."[142]

First, Vaccine Court has likely paid out close to $3 billion dollars as of autumn 2015. Second, had 75 percent of the 5,400 cases—4,050 of them—paid out $500,000 per case (Vaccine Court cap[143]) for vaccine-injured children, with no punitive damages allowed, the total payout would have been $2.025 billion. That is a "b" as in billion, or 1,000 million dollars times two. Even a billion dollar payout, or far less than half of the petitions, would have bankrupted the system and added a billion dollars to the national debt. But it would have done far greater damage to the confidence of new parents, existing parents, pregnant women, and just about everyone else in the United States when they learned the CDC's sacred cow vaccine program causes autism, tics and other health issues. In losing faith in the government-run, pharmaceutical-driven monolith, the entire vaccine industry would have collapsed.

So it was just easier for the CDC to manipulate the data and pay Poul Thorsen more than $11 million to fund numerous seemingly

---

[141] *The Vaccine Court: The Dark Truth of America's Vaccine Injury Compensation Program*, by Wayne Rohde, Skyhorse Publishing, 2014, 2014, page 5.

[142] Ibid, pg. 149

[143] Wikileaks: Congressional Research Service, Report RL31649, Homeland Security Act of 2002: Tort Liability Provision, Henry Cohen, American Law Division, May 9, 2000, pg. CRS-10.

legitimate studies, than to have the above double collapse of the U.S. vaccine program unfold with the enormous payout.

After Julie Gerberding's summer of the "New Normal"—living with the threat of bioterrorism and with the Iraq War having spun out from a conventional ground assault to asymmetrical warfare of IEDs, car bombs, close quarter combat, and sniper traps—September 2003 was back to business in protecting the mercury god thimerosal.

Eight months after Coleen Boyle drafted and sent Jose Cordero's persuasion letter with the Madsen thimerosal study to the journal *Pediatrics*—or was that Ethics?—the CDC's third desperate attempt to publish the article, after twice being rejected by the more prestigious JAMA and Lancet—the study ran in its September 2003 issue.

News of its publication quickly traveled to Aarhus University where Kreesten Madsen was diligently working on his doctoral thesis on vaccines, MMR, thimerosal, and autism. In an email to Diana Schendel on the study making it in *Pediatrics*, he trivialized the moment and effort put forth by the CDC and Poul Thorsen's NANEA to get the "little paper" published.

In other words, the effort, the years and countless hours, the endless CDC input and strategy sessions, the maneuverings, and the tons of emails, communications, expenses, budget reviews, grant funding, wire transfers from the U.S. to Aarhus University, and travel by CDC Drs. Diane Simpson, Paul Stehr-Green, Marshalyn Yeargin-Allsopp, and Diana Schendel, among others, to Denmark—not to mention the millions of dollars the Danish science team received via the CDC's revolving cooperative agreements with NANEA—made that "little paper" big in *their* eyes. It would become one of the six bedrock studies the CDC would use to scaffold its entire argument that vaccines were safe and that thimerosal was no cause for concern, despite the skyrocketing autism rates since the early 1990s.

"Thimerosal and the Occurrence of Autism: Negative Ecological Evidence From Danish Population-Based Data," by PhD candidate Kreesten M. Madsen, Marlene B. Lauritsen, Carsten B. Pedersen,

Poul Thorsen, Anne-Marie Plesner, Peter H. Andersen and Preben B. Mortensen, was published by *Pediatrics*, Volume 112 No. 3, September 2003. It came out on September 1st.

The big "little paper" was a mere two pages long with a cover and fourth page and just fifteen references. Was this worth the years in backtesting data, numerous permutations, and costs that had to approach if not exceed $1 million?

In my June 27, 2015 email with the study's principal investigator, Kreesten Madsen wrote that "Carsten Pedersen was the statistician" on the study. But Pedersen, who worked at Denmark's National Centre for Register-Based Research, University of Aarhus, was never on the email chain between Madsen and the CDC's Coleen Boyle and Diana Schendel, and certainly not part of those CDC doctors directing Madsen or Thorsen to omit the 2001 data from the Danish Health Registries. And since Kreesten Madsen wasn't part of that decision—though Poul Thorsen certainly would have known about it being with Diana Schendel—he confessed he didn't know who called that shot but admitted that the data was indeed left out. He finished by writing to me:

"Again. It is easy to redo the study. It was based on all publicly available registries. Would be nice to see the study redone!"[144] And it has since been redone by Mark Blaxill and Brian Hooker, among other highly educated professionals who are parents of autistic children and want answers on a deliberately opaque CDC process to protect thimerosal and ensure that vaccine production accelerates and doesn't get interrupted by protests from concerned citizens.

In the months and year after the publication of the thimerosal study, many parents from the U.S. autism community began to look at the "little paper." They examined the data, inspected the study's design criteria, checked how the health coding had changed in Denmark during the 1990s, and saw many problems with it that go far beyond leaving the 2001 Danish data out of the statistician's analysis.

---

[144] Email June 27, 2015: Dr. K. M. Madsen to James O. Grundvig.

Perhaps worse than the CDC directing the Danes to omit the 2001 data to skew the study's final results to flatten the data was the charge Kreesten Madsen told over a telephone interview that took place on June 23, 2015.

Madsen said with some burning emotion that "Poul Thorsen was scientifically incompetent. On my MMR study and the thimerosal study, he didn't do any work. Not even during the internal final review process before we submitted it. I was pissed. . . . I brought that to the attention of my superiors at Aarhus University that Thorsen didn't do any work on the study, and they told me to be quiet about it. That pissed me off."

Well, Madsen's supervisor back in the day at Aarhus University was Jørn Olsen. Today, Dr. Olsen is a professor at Aarhus University, Department of Public Health, Dept. of Epidemiology. He also is the principal investigator, leading a team of six Danish scientists at the Center for Longitudinal Studies: Institute of Education, London University: Danish National Birth Cohort. Since graduation from Aarhus University in the 1970s with both a MD and PhD, Jørn Olsen has become a prodigious author and coauthor on more than 400 peer-reviewed epidemiology and, lately, environmental studies, papers, and text books. From 2005–2008, Dr. Jørn Olsen was president of the International Epidemiology Association (IEA),[145] and in 2006 he joined UCLA's School of Public Health, Southern California Injury Prevention Program.

"Jørn Olsen, MD, PhD, is Professor and Chair of the Dept. of Epidemiology, School of Public Health, UCLA. He came to UCLA from Denmark in 2006 where he was head of the Danish Epidemiology Science Centre and was Principal Investigator of the Danish National Birth Cohort, a study among 100,000 pregnant women and their children. The aim of this study is to examine early determinants of

---

[145] http://ieaweb.org/about-iea/history/past-presidents/

health in a cohort that will be followed from conception to death (www.DNBC.DK)."[146]

Jørn Olsen clearly has a sterling international reputation in the science field of epidemiology. His reputation appears above reproach. But as the lead supervisor to Kreesten Madsen during the MMR and thimerosal studies at AU, was it Jørn Olsen who shielded Poul Thorsen doing "no work" on those studies, getting his name on them against Vancouver Protocol? Was it Jørn Olsen who recognized the value of Thorsen as the moneyman from the CDC and needed to protect the U.S. agency's vaccine program? And as a consultant around that time for the U.S. NIH, was Olsen influenced by the inner relationships between the FDA, CDC, NIH, Denmark's SSI, and Aarhus University to tell Madsen to look the other way on Thorsen, the apparent slouch and "incompetent scientist"?

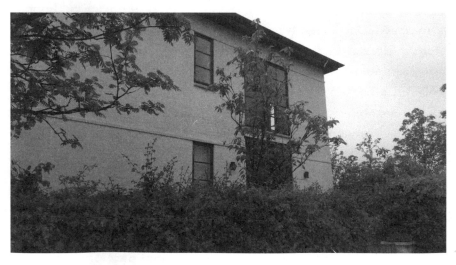

James O. Grundvig

House where Poul Thorsen moved his research group NANEA off campus in Aarhus University around 2004.

---

[146] http://www.ph.ucla.edu/sciprc/Templates/BIOS/11_bio_jorn.htm

One other Danish scientist, Mads Melbye, was the second supervisor to PhD candidate student Kreesten Madsen. Dr. Melbye, Madsen, Thorsen, and Diana Schendel, among others, would share coauthor bylines on several studies between 2002 and 2005. It could have been Mads Melbye, who today runs Denmark's cutting edge BioBank at SSI, who told Madsen to keep quiet on Poul Thorsen lack of involvement.

If the allegations are proven to be true I should learn by summer's end. In an email to me on Monday, July 13, 2015, Allan Flyvbjerg, Dean of Health at Aarhus University, had agreed to examine that claim, among others, writing: "I'm presently at summer vacation, as is the administrative staff I need to address the various elements of your inquiry in a meticulous way. We will get back to you in the first half of August."[147]

The first charge, in which Poul Thorsen "did no work" on the key Danish studies for the CDC, goes against the Vancouver Protocol on reference papers, or more precisely, the "Uniform Requirements for Manuscripts Submitted to Biomedical Journals" by the International Committee of Medical Journal Editors. And two of the main points of the Vancouver Protocol on authors' credits are:

> Third, authors sending manuscripts to a participating journal should not try to prepare them in accordance with the publication style of that journal but should follow the Uniform Requirements.
>
> Authors must also follow the instructions to authors in the journal as to what topics are suitable for that journal and the types of papers that may be submitted—for example, original articles, reviews, or case reports. In addition, the journal's instructions are likely to contain other requirements unique to that journal, such as the number of copies of a manuscript

---

[147] Email July 13, 2015: Dr. Allan Flyvbjerg, Dean of Health at Aarhus University, to James O. Grundvig.

that are required, acceptable languages, length of articles, and approved abbreviations.[148]

If Aarhus University does prove that Poul Thorsen didn't do any "substantial" work on the studies, against international journal standards, then not only does his name need to be stricken from those studies, but it also brings into question whether those studies were published under false pretenses to begin with—as there is a "conflicts of interest" section that all study authors need to fill out for full disclosure—then the "bedrock" study needs to be retracted, plain and simple.

On Dr. Olsen's EpiBlog for IEA website on Conflicts of Interest, he opened:

Epidemiology often addresses research problems where results have implications for many people. Research of this nature has to be of good quality and conclusions should reflect validity and sources of bias in a fair manner, not influenced by any other "outside" factors. Epidemiologists with conflicts of interest— "defined as a set of circumstances that creates a risk that professional judgement or actions regarding a primary interest will be unduly influenced by a secondary interest"—should declare these conflicts when they seek funding, report their results, provide legal opinions, and in scientific correspondence. We also recognize that conflicts of interest go further than financial conflicts; political views, prior trust in the hypothesis and even a sense of ownership of the hypothesis all play a role together with many other factors, including family and other relationships. For these reasons data should always be available for others to reanalyze.[149]

---

[148] Vancouver Protocol, the Fifth Addition (1997), pg. 1.

[149] http://ieaweb.org/conflicts-of-interest/ - by Jørn Olsen, EpiBlog, February 12, 2014.

If Jørn Olsen stands by his written word and was the one who told Kreesten Madsen to keep quiet on Poul Thorsen's out-to-lunch approach to scientific research, because of the grant money Thorsen was raking in from the CDC, then Olsen should have no problem stating that he was the supervisor who snuffed Madsen's complaint, not in the name of science, but in the name of commerce.

Whatever damage all of the data manipulation might do to the CDC and its Drs. Coleen Boyle, Diane Simpson, Jose Cordero, and Diana Schendel (who was now working an as epidemiologist research professor on autism at Aarhus University), to Poul Thorsen and to everyone else involved, it should not deter AU's Dean of Health from doing the right thing.

In speaking with another source at Aarhus University, on the condition of anonymity, she said that when Poul Thorsen was a professor lecturing in class during the early 2000s, he wasn't very good at it. "Thorsen wasn't a good teacher. Poul and three other professors (including Kreesten Madsen) at Aarhus University taught a class of 160 students. That class was split equally with 40 students in each class. I was one of those students," she explained. "A week into the semester, the other professors each ended up with 50 students, since they were free to go to any of the four classes. As that happened, poor Poul had only eleven students left to teach. He wasn't a good professor."

Apparently Poul Thorsen was a better schmoozer, lover, and grant-money raiser than scientist or teacher.

With three-quarters of the students changing classes on account of Poul Thorsen's poor lecturing skills and inability to convey or articulate lessons in his class, Kreesten Madsen never thought highly of Dr. Thorsen as a person or scientist. During the phone interview, Dr. Madsen said, "Poul was a lousy scientist. He was scientifically incompetent. But he was bringing in the money from the CDC. As far as I am concerned, I wouldn't buy a used car from Thorsen."

His dislike, bordering on disrespect, for Poul Thorsen can be verified by Dr. Madsen's actions. After earning his PhD in 2004, he distanced himself from Thorsen, NANEA, and the CDC. He would spend the next three years at Aarhus University doing research and coauthoring a handful of studies with Dr. Jørn Olsen, Mads Melbye, and a few others before he left to SSI.

When Kreesten Madsen left Arhus University for good in 2007 or so, he headed to Sjaelland, Denmark's main island where the capital city of Copenhagen is located more than three hours by car or train from the town of Aarhus. Over the next several years, Kreesten Madsen went to work for three pharmaceutical research companies: Novo Nordisk A/S, just outside Copenhagen; Nycomed, to the west of the city; and Alk Alebello, in the capital region, before choosing to become a medical doctor consultant in the Hovedstaden region.[150]

Most likely a good athlete in his youth, Kreesten Madsen was busy before the Danish summer holiday in July, both and work and coordinating a triathlon event in late June, he told me at the end of our telephone interview.

More than half of the original two-dozen doctors, scientists, students, and staff that made up the 2002 NANEA team, which I screen-scraped from the Web, remain working today at Aarhus University in some research, professor or scientific capacity. Not Madsen. He left Aarhus as if to get as many miles away from Poul Thorsen as possible. And even though Aarhus University's then-managing director Jørgen Jørgensen exiled Thorsen from the university in 2010, Poul managed to import Diana Schendel to Aarhus University in 2013 after a twenty-one year career at the CDC. By 2014, Dr. Schendel became a full-time faculty member at AU in the Department of Public Health, Dept. of Epidemiology; the Dept. of Economics and Business Economics, CIRRAU—Centre for Integrated Register-based Research; and NCRR—National Centre for Register-based Research.[151]

---

[150] https://dk.linkedin.com/pub/kreesten-meldgaard-madsen/5/143/184

[151] http://pure.au.dk/portal/en/persons/diana-schendel(2163da2c-859c-46e1-b464-d1c36b753696).html

But beyond the major flaws, ethics violations, and foibles that made up Poul Thorsen's character and his inability to teach students well or effectively or be competent enough for input on serious scientific studies, Kreesten Madsen's thimerosal study was flawed beyond Thorsen's credit for authorship and the missing 2001 data.

Mark Blaxill, a tireless writer, researcher, and editor, today with Age of Autism and back in 2000 was the director at SafeMinds, had gotten his hands on an "embargoed" copy of *Pediatrics*' soon-to-be-published Madsen thimerosal study.

Armed with an undergraduate degree from Princeton University and a MBA from Harvard, Mark Blaxill had authored and co-authored nine studies from 2002 to 2008. He also wrote and presented speeches at autism-vaccine rallies in Washington, D.C., presented his findings during Congressional hearings,[152] and did his own deep dive into the Danish studies and the linkages between the CDC and the Danish scientists involved, including Poul Thorsen, Kreesten Madsen, and Diana Schendel, as well as the incestuous ties with Danish vaccine policy and manufacturer Statens Serum Institute.

In an email, Mark Blaxill wrote how he responded to the thimerosal study in a detailed brief one day after its publication.

"I first saw the embargoed copy of the paper on Wednesday, August 27th. A reporter from the Associated Press had received it from the journal and was asking SafeMinds for comments and she shared it with us. I spent much of the Labor day weekend working on the critique. We finalized it by Monday (and sent the response to the AP reporter) and released the analysis along with a press release on Tuesday September 2nd.

"There was a frenzy of activity around then.

"I had taken a sabbatical from BCG that summer and was very focused on the autism-thimerosal debate as it was breaking. I was

---

[152] http://www.ageofautism.com/2012/12/safeminds-mark-blaxill-testimony-at-autism-hearing.html

working through the final phases of preparing an article I wrote the for International Journal of Toxicology (Holmes, Blaxill and Haley, 2003), there was a draft rebuttal to another Danish study that I was working on as well (American Journal of Preventive Medicine, 2003, Stehr-Green et al), there were rebuttals to Nelson and Bauman's *Pediatrics* article and Pichichero's Lancet article, a draft of my epidemiology that was published in Public Health Reports in 2004 and the ongoing work on the Evidence of Harm project.

"The Madsen *Pediatrics* publication came out in the middle of all this; looking back, it was all a bit of a blur.

"The most important insight I've had on the study since this critique was the observation of all the institutional linkages [of which Thorsen was a part] surrounding the Danish papers. I did a social network analysis of the author network sometime in early 2004 and even tried to submit an article for publication in 2005."[153]

In a letter to the editor titled "Concerns Continue Over Mercury and Autism" in the *American Journal of Preventative Medicine*, Blaxill defended his analysis of the Madsen thimerosal study in a public tête-a-tête with CDC's Paul Stehr-Green, writing:

Their autism cases account for a fraction of the autism population. The large majority of autism cases are found in outpatient populations. Yet, the analyses in Sweden (exclusively) and Denmark (for two thirds of the study period) rely on inpatient populations. One recent Danish study revealed that 93% of autistic records were for outpatients. Clearly, the small remaining group of inpatient registrations has little value in trend assessment.[154]

---

[153] Email July 19, 2015: From Mark Blaxill, Editor at Large Age of Autism, to James O. Grundvig.

[154] Letters to the Editor, Concerns Continue Over Mercury and Autism, *American Journal of Preventative Medicine*, 2004; 26(1).

So either the CDC's Coleen Boyle or Diana Schendel gave explicit direction to Madsen and Thorsen's team to omit the 2001 data from the Danish Health Registries, which would have shown a leveling off or a decline in autism rates in Denmark. By 2003, the study's data and analysis had become so bastardized it excluding other critical data.

Mark Blaxill wrote and published a more detailed paper—the same four page length with no cover sheet and similar fourteen references as Madsen's Thimerosal Study—stating:

"Autism counts were first based on hospitalized, inpatient records and then changed in the middle of the study period to add in outpatient records. This new outpatient registry was introduced in 1995."[155]

Beyond the Danish fish stew of cooking the data several different ways, is the thimerosal Material Safety Data Sheet (MSDS) from the patent holder and manufacturer Eli Lilly that is used today.

A MSDS sheet is used in chemical manufacturing operations and processing plants, laboratories, and construction sites where special chemicals, substances, and materials are used and where a worker may be exposed to the chemical. Onsite there would be a MSDS book that, when EMS arrives to treat and take an ailing person to a hospital, would ride with that patient to the emergency room so that the physician can read through the manufacturer's literature to see how certain chemicals or compounds could impact human health, cause harm, and how to treat symptoms.

From Eli Lilly's own 1999–2000 MSDS sheet on thimerosal, key insights read:

- **Chemical Family:** Organomercurial salt
- Thimerosal contains 49.6% w/w organically-bound mercury.

---

[155] "Danish Thimerosal-Autism Study in Pediatrics: Misleading and Uninformative on Autism-Mercury Link," by Mark Blaxill, Director SafeMinds, September 2, 2003.

- **Exposure Guidelines:** Thimerosal—No known occupational exposure limits established.
- **Primary Physical and Health Hazards:** Skin Permeable. Toxic. Mutagen. Irritant (eyes).
- Allergen. Nervous System and Reproductive Effects.
- **Caution Statement:** Thimerosal may enter the body through the skin, is toxic, alters genetic material, may be irritating to the eyes, and causes allergic reactions. Effects of exposure may include numbness of extremities, fetal changes, decreased offspring survival, and lung tissue changes.
- **Effects of Overexposure:** Topical allergic dermatitis has been reported. Thimerosal contains mercury. Mercury poisoning may occur and topical hypersensitivity reactions may be seen
- Early signs of mercury poisoning in adults are nervous system effects, including narrowing of the visual field and numbness in the extremities.
- Exposure to mercury in utero and in children may cause mild to severe mental retardation and mild to severe motor coordination impairment.
- Based on animal data, may be irritating to the eyes.
- **Spills:** This material is a mercury compound which are CERCLA Hazardous Substances and SARA 313 Toxic Chemicals.
- **Incompatibility:** May react with strong oxidizing agents (e.g., peroxides, permanganates, nitric acid, etc.).
- **Hazardous Decomposition:** May emit toxic mercury fumes when heated to decomposition.
- **Oral:** Rat, median lethal dose 73 mg/kg, reduced activity, drooping eyelids, weakness.
- **Intravenous:** Rat, median lethal dose estimated greater than 45 mg/kg, mortality.
- **Chronic Exposure** Thimerosal is a mercuric compound. Toxicity data for thimerosal and mercury are presented.

- **Reproduction:** Thimerosal—Decreased offspring survival. Mercury—Changes in sperm production, decreased offspring survival, and offspring nervous system effects including mild to severe mental retardation and motor coordination impairment.
- **EC Classification:**
- **T+** (Very Toxic)
- **N** (Dangerous for the Environment)
- **Medical Conditions Aggravated by Exposure:** Hypersensitivity to mercury.[156]


When reading through the eight-page MSDS on thimerosal, which is twice as long as typical MSDS sheets on paints, mastics, primers, polymers, and caustic chemicals that I have reviewed during my years in the construction industry, many things jump out—all of them bad, all of them warning signs, and all of them adverse to the human body, especially to newborn babies and vulnerable pregnant women.

Most alarming is the "motor coordination impairment," a clear sign of tics and part of the autism spectrum, the two European Union (EU) classifications of "very toxic" and "dangerous for the environment"; and lastly a pre-existing medical condition, genetic flaw or susceptibility to "hypersensitivity to mercury."

Nowhere on Eli Lilly's MSDS sheet does it state a safe, minute amount. Quite the opposite. Remember; former U.S. Senator Dick Armey went out of his way to protect both the manufacturer and thimerosal itself, including the reputation of ex-President George H. W. Bush who "was a board member of the Eli Lilly Co., which holds the patent for thimerosal. White House Budget Planning Director Mitch Daniels worked as a top executive at Lilly. The company's president, Sidney Taurel, is a member of the Homeland Security Advisory

---

[156] Eli Lilly and Company, Material Safety Data Sheet, "Thimerosal." Effective Date Dec. 22, 1999.

Council, and is closely tied to President Bush, according to the report. Scores of lawsuits filed against Lilly by the families of thimerosal victims have yielded no results."[157]

And then Lilly got full immunity from prosecution by the Armey Rider.

---

[157] Wikileaks: Ankara Media Reaction Report Thursday, August 18, 2005, Press Briefing on "*Vaccine Crisis* in the U.S."

# OTHER PEOPLE'S MONEY

People, especially peers, grew tired of listening to Poul Thorsen's self-important blather on NANEA and how his research group was going to change the world, and former lecture students and his main study cog Kreesten Meldgaard Madsen left NANEA by the end of 2004. The Dane, whose name translates to the "Son of Thor," hired a bunch of low wage groupies, many of them as "contract workers," not full-time employees with benefits, while overcharging the CDC through its cooperative agreement at much higher rates for more senior-type positions.

The first, innocuous-looking fraud became overshadowed by the outright twenty-two counts Thorsen was charged with by the U.S. Dept. of Justice (DOJ). But the "contract workers" label would eventually get those young, cheap, naive employees in trouble with the Danish tax authority when the house of cards of NANEA began to crumble in early 2009. With Thorsen skimming money through various CDC bank accounts he held, on top of making the differential between fees and what he actually paid out to lesser talent and experienced employees, he was clearly abusing the cooperative agreement he signed with the CDC. Thorsen probably breached that as far back as 2004, and ethically, at bare minimum, with the CDC and Aarhus University. He made profits above and beyond the market rate overhead and profit fees that are typical to government-funded work that's allowed to be charged.

The ruse works like this. Say a worker with the label Project Manager (PM) has a fee that can be charged at $125 per hour. Add 20% overhead for benefit costs, such as mobile phones, computers, and insurance premiums, and the hourly rate jumps to $150/hour. Thorsen turns around and pays his low-level, NANEA non-employees—they are contractors—$20/hour and the half dozen interns who work there at half that rate or even nothing at all, except for having a spiffy-looking research job on their resume. Other employees like Madsen might have been billed to the CDC or Aarhus University's Dept. of Epidemiology. Either way, NANEA should have been a cash cow, a money machine, or a farm with an endless amount of real estate to grow. It used Danish citizen's own personal health data for free, without giving anything in return—without making a single product, such as software, a mobile app, or a database, without designing a new analysis or solution, and without ever developing any intellectual property at all.

As an office engineer, change management engineer, and project manager I have worked on projects of scale with the Federal Heavy Highway Commission, the states Departments of Transportation in Pennsylvania, New Jersey and the City of New York on heavy highway renovations; the Port Authority of New Jersey/New York on the JFK/ American Airlines project; Baruch College "Vertical Campus" with the Dormitory Authority of the State of New York (DASNY); various public school projects for the NYC School Construction Authority; and the first LEED-Gold condominium in NY State history with the Battery Park City Authority, a quasi-state entity. Over my 25+ year engineering-construction career, I have seen, monitored, exposed, negotiated, and tracked orders of this ruse over and again.

Clearly, neither the CDC nor Aarhus University had any quality control in place as a system of checks and balances on Poul Thorsen, master manipulator. And even though language was written into the cooperative agreements that allowed audits of bookkeeping to be reviewed each year by the Center for Disease Control, if Diana Schendel was the scientist who was supposed to keep an eye on that workflow, she most likely kept an eye on Thorsen's zipper instead.

Exit Ib Terp. In November 2004, Ib won the election to become Brøndby's mayor beginning January 1, 2005. With Mr. Terp out of the picture, Poul Thorsen had no one at the CDC, Aarhus University, the Danish Medical Research Council, Statens Serum Institut, or NANEA to watch over him to make sure that bills were paid, payroll was met, and that the temptation to steal research money pledged to autism, alcohol, and cerebral palsy research wouldn't go missing.

Much like the swelling of the U.S. housing bubble unfolding at the same time, money was available everywhere. It was cheap, with the banks pushing credits and loans like drug dealers peddling designer meds. Poul Thorsen stood at the perfect time, at the ideal intersection with no one watching his actions. Partially set up by Ib Terp's exit, having a steamy affair with CDC scientist Diana Schendel, hiring young "yes" people to work at NANEA and believe his big words and grand vision of NANEA becoming a global leader in scientific research, and chasing off Kreesten Madsen—who might have been the only one to expose Thorsen's fraud earlier had he stuck around at Aarhus University instead of work for the pharmaceutical companies in Copenhagen—Poul Thorsen was one lucky thief in the making.

There was no one and nothing to stop him.

# I 6

# CASH AND BURN

Poul Thorsen had to have loved his arrangement with the CDC.

What was not to love?

The CDC, his golden calf, had brought the obscure research scientist notoriety—at a young age for his profession—to his conservative-in-behavior homeland of Denmark. It gave him a girlfriend in Diana Schendel; they shared the same affinity and interest in the field of epidemiology, from childhood disorders (autism) and diseases (cerebral palsy) to the health, elasticity, and susceptibility of the vagina.

And for him, Dr. Schendel was the E–ZPass lane. She was a direct conduit to the stars, with access to the constellation of executives of the U.S. healthcare agency who were in dire need to drum up answers to keep its bloated vaccine program from imploding and to keep in check the crazed parents of the autism epidemic, and were willing to pay for it all. Add flashes of American wealth and freedom, combined with the potent brew of capitalism with billboards and advertisements streaming dreams of sex and riches into his mind everyday—it all must have struck a chord deep inside Thorsen. It hit a nerve. It awakened his heart, soul, and libido. It lit a fire that flashed images of fame, wealth, power, houses, scantily clad women, sports cars, yachts, and glory.

Yes, glory.

Poul Thorsen relished the idea, the dream of seeing his name in lights, on the big screen like Hollywood, on the studies (on some of which he did little to no work), and one day in books, magazines, and TV shows that would profile him and his illustrious career for the world. Once he solved the CDC's problems with the vats and pools of Danish health data, he could export NANEA's business around the world and grow evermore wealthy and famous in the process. And if he did it right, he might become the best-known Danish scientist outside of Scandinavia, surpassing Denmark's thirteen Nobel Laureates in medicine and science.[158]

Aarhus University had its own Nobel Laureate in Jens Christian Skou,[159] the 1997 co-winner in chemistry for his discovery of a special enzyme function that "pumps sodium out of cells, while pumping potassium into cells. It has antiporter-like activity but is not actually an antiporter since both molecules are moving against their concentration gradient."[160]

But Poul Thorsen was no Nobel Laureate, nor anywhere near the same plateau, let alone planet, that Jens Skou occupied. The only thing Thorsen would ever discover was how to exploit the needy CDC, which long before the autism epidemic of 2000 had become politically corrupt in its search to find "no link" between the dioxins of Agent Orange, the flights of Operation Hand, and the U.S. Army troops on the ground.

A victory for Monsanto, Dow Chemical, other vendors in the Agent Orange supply chain, the Reagan White House, and the CDC, in particular Coleen Boyle who would end up being promoted over and over again. Impervious Boyle rose at Teflon CDC.

---

[158] https://en.wikipedia.org/wiki/List_of_Nobel_laureates_by_country#Denmark

[159] https://en.wikipedia.org/wiki/Jens_Christian_Skou

[160] https://en.wikipedia.org/wiki/Na%2B/K%2B-ATPase

More opportunist than scientist, Thorsen was a mere visiting foreign scientist arriving at the right time in the right country with the right agency during its biggest crisis with the autism epidemic fanning flames of fear through the cities, towns, and communities of America. All Poul had to do was show up and play along to leverage the situation and vulnerabilities of the CDC. Sleeping with the help was a bonus. The Dane tuned into and played off the desperate fears of the CDC's higher-ups that the rise of the debilitating neurological disorder could derail the U.S. vaccine machine, which would slice into the pharmaceutical giants' bottom line. We're talking about billions of dollars of industry revenue, with billions more in profits, stocks, and shareholder value.

Without knowing it at first, Poul Thorsen stood at the fulcrum of the autism epidemic and the U.S. immunization program. Like two children on a seesaw, he observed it wouldn't take much to tip the balance to one side of the other. By the turn of the millennium he read the signs on the horizon marking vaccines as unsafe with a bulls-eye.

As the CDC scrambled internally to find the data to explain how thimerosal was not the cause in the sharp rise of autism incidence in modern, educated countries that had banned the mercury preservative, U.S. Senator Dick Armey used balls and politics to insert the "Lilly Rider" into the Homeland Security Act of 2002 in the twelfth hour to protect the producer of thimerosal from tort liability. What was left? Whatever it was, Poul Thorsen must have viewed the Chinese fire drill at the CDC, with executives scurrying about, as if he were on the deck of the Titanic with half-full lifeboats being launched—a golden opportunity to fast track his career while bringing both scientific fame and fortune to his medical career back in Denmark. From there, he could consult and secure grant money from many different agencies in Denmark and abroad, as well as foundations and non-profits.

Thorsen would align himself with the right names in the right seats of power in the Danish science, medical research, and university ecosystem to cement his reputation as a problem solver of the highest order. He knew raising grant money was a long, laborious process for many scientists. The fact that Thorsen could pull in more than one million U.S. dollars from the CDC per year must have made his peers and superiors in Denmark think that he had the Midas touch. He sure thought so.

The CDC reciprocated by giving the Danish scientist— "incompetent" in the words of Kreesten Madsen—a government agency email address and allowed Thorsen to open several bank accounts at the CDC Federal Credit Union, which had a grand total of three branches with a very finite clientele base. In the end, Thorsen would have more accounts than the bank had branches.

From the bank's own website, membership is allowed "if you meet any of the following eligibility requirements:

- If you live, work, worship, attend school, or volunteer in portions of DeKalb, Fulton, or Gwinnett Counties.
- You are a present employee (or family member of an employee) of: The Centers for Disease Control and Prevention, its subsidiaries, affiliates or contractors."[161]

Evidently, this would be no obstacle for the foreign visiting scientist since the CDC gave him the go ahead to open a government credit union bank account under the "affiliates or contractors" label. There, the CDC made a huge gaffe. It allowed Poul Thorsen to invoice the CDC under his cooperative agreement, and since he was the principal investigator for NANEA under the Danish Medical Research Council, he was in charge of disbursements. Once the monies were sent overseas, all the alleged thief had to do was create a backdoor to

---

[161] https://www.cdcfcu.com/Online-Services/Join.aspx

send an invoice back to the States in one of five CDC Federal Credit
Union bank accounts he controlled.

How hard would it have been for Thorsen to invoice Aarhus
University? Not hard at all. In fact, it was damn easy to complete
the boomerang in funds. All Poul needed was CDC letterhead—he
could have gotten that during his numerous visits to CDC executive offices, or when Diana Schendel was asleep, or even been given
a ream during one of his numerous visits to its Atlanta headquarters
over the years. Then he would need a name, a close approximation
of that person's signature, and an email address to send the invoice
and another to receive it in the accounting department at AU, which
in turn would ask Poul Thorsen to approve payment. The Dane was
in total control of the process. And with Ib Terp out the door from
NANEA to become mayor of Brøndby in late 2005, there was no one
there to double-check his books or develop and monitor an audit trail
of monies in and monies out. So he decided to start the fraud early in
February—a month after the ink dried with the renewal of the 2004
CDC-NANEA cooperative agreement. Why not? Why wait longer?

The CDC and United States were flush with cash, as Atlanta built a
half dozen new luxury office buildings and high-rise condominiums,
average Americans were flipping houses in Las Vegas and California,
and Europeans were investing in condos in Miami to use as a second
vacation home.

From the court case filed on April 13, 2011, known as *United States
of America vs. Poul Thorsen*, the opening of thirteen wire fraud counts
by the Grand Jury read:

> 1. Beginning on a date unknown, but at least by in or about
> February 2004, and continuing until in or about February 2010,
> in the Northern District of Georgia and elsewhere the defend-
> ant, POUL THORSEN, aided and abetted by others known
> and unknown to the Grand Jury, did knowingly devise and
> intend to devise a scheme and artifice to defraud, and to obtain

money and property by means of materially false and fraudulent pretenses, representations,and promises, and by omission of
material facts.[162]

With no business partner per se after Ib Terp's departure in an
election year, and no internal audits or controls in place at the
CDC, Aarhus University, or Odense University Hospital with either
Thorsen or NANEA, the Dane was free to do what he wanted with
all that grant money, including siphoning it off in large chunks if he
so wished. There literally was nothing to stop him.

So perfect was the climate for theft that it had to be too much
for Poul Thorsen to resist. The insulated, above the treetops view of
the CDC and its problems had to empower him and so, seeing the
golden opportunity some years before the alleged fraud took place,
he immersed himself deeper into the culture of the CDC. His affair
with Diana Schendel moved beyond the bed sheets and strolls on the
beaches in summer near Aarhus and extended into their professional
lives in the forty studies—and counting—they worked on together
in some capacity. Publishing the studies with "Lady Diana" and her
CDC colleagues cemented his relationship with the agency permanently—or so he anticipated.

Like unqualified homebuyers from valet car parkers at the casinos
to strippers from the Las Vegas Strip, making $40,000 to $50,000 a
year could secure a $1 million, 30-year, variable rate mortgage with
no money down. Thorsen must have thought he had won the lottery.
And he had, for a while. But like all lottery winners or gamblers on a
hot streak, the earnings that come with winning eventually taper off,
stop abruptly, or reverse course like a losing streak.

For many Americans, however, who needed only to look back five
short years to view the burst of the hyperinflated dot-com bubble,

---

[162] Case 1:11-cr-00194-UNA, Doc 1, Filed 4/13/11, "USA vs. Poul Thorsen" by
U.S. District Attorney Sally Quillian Yates, pg. 1.

Poul Thorsen overlooked the ceiling of the CDC's own billions of dollars of annual budget. He must have thought the law of gravity didn't apply to economics, global markets, and governments. Well, it does. And with the axiom "what goes up, must come down," there will always be the terminal velocity of free fall the faster and steeper one climbs.

Dr. Thorsen's research group NANEA was never positioned for when a market correction would one day emerge. But clearly, whatever his shortcomings as a scientist, those same foibles didn't serve him well in his business operations. If anyone could have checked his ego and kept him in balance, that person would have been Diana Schendel, who, when the time and mood was right, had her boy by the balls. But dear Diana had her own two failed marriages: she needed to continue to keep distance in her life. And not coming from the hyper-competitive world of business—the private sector—driven by the winds of free markets, she didn't have the wherewithal to tug on the string of that kite that was Poul Thorsen, aloft, free, soaring, uplifted by his vision of NANEA, and pull him back to earth. Like many people Poul had sold himself and the perception of his expertise and scientific success to, Schendel didn't bother to tether him in place. That was her personal gaffe, as she would become guilty by association and a lot more.

In the U.S. DOJ, the Southern District of Georgia indictment of Poul Thorsen listed twenty-two counts of wire fraud (13) and money laundering (9), covering the period from May 30, 2006, to October 29, 2008. The latter date was one month after the fixed income bubble burst and the Great Recession started. Maybe the date of October 29th could have hinted how bad the economy was going to tank. The Vegas valets and strippers certainly knew. Money dried up in desert pools. Big time gamblers disappeared as the stock market cratered, and housing prices imploded down into a massive sinkhole of debt. Too many middle class Americans were unemployed, looking for new jobs, underwater with their mortgages, crushed by outstanding credit card debt, and had too few savings and a 401-K retirement plan that went south along with the rest of investments.

With no safe havens left, Poul Thorsen would tap the mother lode one more time. But even he felt the cold wind of financial gravity shake his confidence.

U.S. Attorney Yates's indictment stated that "before, on or around February 2004" Poul Thorsen launched his scheme to defraud the CDC, Aarhus University, and even his own startup research group NANEA.

There has been no word from the Federal Bureau of Investigation (FBI) about what other criminal acts Thorsen might have committed during the year and a half leading up to the first money laundering charge; or from the U.S. DOJ after four long years of failing to extradite the Danish scientist to learn the full scope of his schemes; or from Poul Thorsen through his Aarhus-based attorney Jan Schneider, who didn't respond to requests to be interviewed or offer to co-write Thorsen's biography.

Like a child at the cookie jar or a teenager dipping into his father's bottle of vodka, Thorsen only took a little at a time. Wait and see. No reaction? Take a little more. Like a drug user trying to learn both the potency of a drug and his limits of absorbing it at the same time, Poul Thorsen took this tried-and-true method of human experimentation to become a white-collar criminal, taking the first step to skimming profits or milking a system like Ponzi master Bernie Madoff.

The first item Poul Thorsen purchased was a 2004 Audi S4 Avant Quattro, which was listed in the DOJ indictment.[163] He probably bought the V8 high-performance vehicle, which took premium unleaded gasoline only, with a small to no down payment—as it was the rise of free credit and the U.S. housing bubble—and financed the vehicle with a three-to five-year loan. Off the top he probably siphoned money from NANEA's coffers. He did it monthly in small amounts. A couple thousand dollars would be more than enough to

---

[163] Ibid, pg. 8.

cover the monthly payments for an Audi Quattro, fuel, service, main-
tenance, and parking if needed. Perhaps he didn't need parking since
Diana Schendel could have used the vehicle when he was back in
Denmark and park it at her home outside of Atlanta.

When he made a dozen or so payments, quietly skimming a little more each month from NANEA, Poul Thorsen became more
emboldened, more daring. As both the head of NANEA and the
principal investigator for all of the studies, even if he wasn't the true
PI or his name wasn't in that lead position of a particular study, like
Bernie Madoff, Thorsen probably kept two sets of books: one for the
investors and authorities, the other for himself. Since he was a scientist
who raised grant money from charities, non-profits, state agencies,
and foundations, he sold names, his connections, and his backing by
the CDC, blessed by various executives there.

One day in one meeting, Thorsen would name-drop Bob Chen,
at the time the chief of Vaccine Safety at the CDC's National
Immunization Program. The next day he would use Dr. Coleen Boyle,
Queen of Agent Orange. And then at the next meeting, the Dane
would wrangle out Jose Cordero, the Don Quixote of letter writing
Such a salesman, Poul Thorsen would always sell three studies ahead
with more rainbow promises to follow. Finances of NANEA didn't
matter to him. Why would it? He believed he would never have to
show how he dispersed the grant money or ever show either set of
books to anyone; the money tap would always be open.

That, of course, was pure fantasy, a detachment from how the real
world works.

Thorsen, like Schendel, had never worked one day of his life in
the private sector. And because of that, he didn't understand that the
insular world outside governments, foundations, institutions, and universities was a wolf-eat-dog world. He would never have survived,
other than selling used cars on a back alley lot just as Kreesten Madsen
so aptly observed a dozen years ago. Poul Thorsen knew there was
no system of internal controls in place that would look under the

hood of NANEA. But then he knew little, or didn't care to know, about the changing seats of power inside governments, and the need for bureaucracy, from time to time, to find, hoist, and flog scapegoats when the tide of public opinion turned against them in a blistering wave of criticism.

The CDC's Dr. Robert T. Chen would become one such fall guy when internal complaints arose that labeled him as lax and unresponsive with other scientists outside the CDC hierarchy. So in December 2004, most likely Director Julie Gerberding had Bob Chen removed from NIP as its lead safety officer to CDC infection safety coordinator, where he had worked for two years. Over the next five years, Bob Chen became the agency's HIV Vaccine and Special Studies team leader—Dr. Gerberding's specialty—before he moved to his current position of medical office, Clinical Trials Team, after she went to Merck to become president of its Vaccine Division in 2009.

For someone who dropped the ball on thimerosal, when he had the chance to do the right thing back when he attended both the aluminum and Simpsonwood meetings in spring 2000, Dr. Chen doubled down and worked in an area that must have confused him at first if the Clinical Trials Team actually tested vaccines on live babies, infants, and children, as opposed to backtesting data the Danish way.

Outside of an agency or university going through a tumultuous year created by change in management, there was no reason for Poul Thorsen to ever suspect that the powers of the CDC or at AU would change their ways and demand something they hadn't asked for for six years: an internal audit under the veil of quality assurance. As long as he, his team, his name, and NANEA made it onto the produced studies, who from the CDC or AU would ever need to inspect his books? No one, he figured.

Through 2005, more than five years running, no one had ever questioned, requested or even hinted at taking a peek into NANEA's books, let alone doing a deep dive into the research group's finances—despite the fact that the annual cooperative agreement allowed for an internal review by either the CDC or AU.

"There have to be accounted for US research grant from the period 2000–2007, but the process will be drawn out again and again. According to chief accountant at Odense University Hospital (OUH) Niels Henning Poulsen is the problem primarily because there has

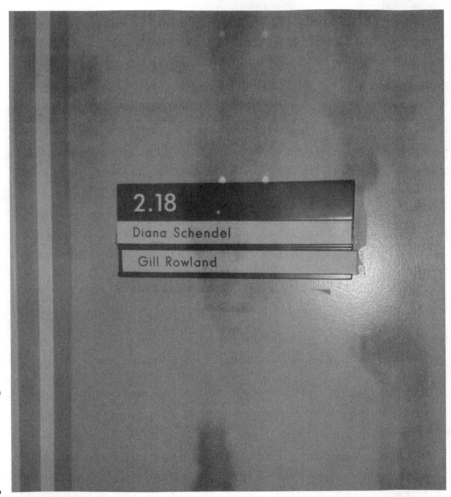

James O. Grundvig

Diana Schendel's nameplate on her office door at Aarhus University.

not been accounted in the research project first seven years, because neither the CDC or the Agency for Science had demanded it."[164]

Poul Bak Thorsen was a research scientist. In his eyes, he was a winner who brought home to Denmark Viking-esque boatloads of cash in U.S. research dollars. Why question that? Well, they didn't. And he assumed they never would.

So it was time for him to up the ante and test the waters again, this time a little more boldly in the deep end of the pool. He set his eyes on a true icon of American freedom: a Harley Davidson motorcycle, the mustang of U.S. roads and highways.

Teflon-protected Poul Thorsen traveled Memorial Day week to Stone Mountain, Georgia. Paul drove thirty minutes southeast from the Centers for Disease of Disease Control headquarters at 1600 Clifton Road near Druid Hills, Atlanta, into the heart of America's racial divide, Stone Mountain, a small town of 5,000-plus residents in DeKalb County.

The town is centered around a mountain that pre-native Americans must have worshipped in ancient times, since it rises by itself like a massive whale breaching the lakes and forestlands. The monument rock has Southern Civil War heroes Davis, Lee, and Jackson chiseled into its massive granite façade.

In 1915, Stone Mountain became the point for the resurgence of the Ku Klux Klan. But like the confederate flag of 2015, which met a swift demise in the wake of the Charleston church massacre, it was Martin Luther King Jr.'s words that resonate today from his "I Have a Dream" speech: "Let freedom ring from Stone Mountain of Georgia."[165]

Thus it was highly improbable that selfish Poul Thorsen knew or cared about any of the history of Stone Mountain, Georgia. His

---

[164] *Danish Researcher in Consumption Trap*, by Lise Richter of www.information. dk, May 23, 2011, pg. 3-4.

[165] http://www.archives.gov/press/exhibits/dream-speech.pdf

eyes were fixated on a 2006 limited edition classic Harley Davidson Screamin' Eagle Fat Boy (FLSTFSE2) motorcycle, not some geologic feature of Civil War remembrance etched in stone. On the day after Memorial Day, Thorsen wrote a personal check from his CDC Federal Credit Union checking account (#3353) in the full amount of $33,994.57.[166]

Poul Thorsen, the tall man with a warm, humorous, insightful personality, didn't pull one over the Harley Davidson salesman who serviced him. Because he didn't need to finance the red Harley, he beat his chest and wrote the full amount on his check, as if he were a millionaire. It was American taxpayer money intended for autism research that bought the sterling motorcycle. And instead of increasing in value, like antique cars in mint condition, Thorsen's Fat Boy motorcycle that held his fat butt depreciated by more than 50 percent in today's open market.[167]

When he finally drove the Harley up past Stone Mountain in search of a new home to live in within a stone's throw from the CDC and Emory University, his underfunded NANEA began to lose steam. Thorsen was sold neither a classic nor a lemon motorcycle, but not a home run either.

Fool's gold would seduce the "incompetent" scientist one more time.

---

[166] Case 1:11-cr-00194-UNA, Doc 1, Filed 4/13/11, "USA vs. Poul Thorsen" by U.S. District Attorney Sally Quillian Yates, pg. 6.

[167] http://www.cycletrader.com/HARLEY--DAVIDSON-FLSTFSE-Screamin... Boy%7C764856244&sort=geo_distance%3Aasc&layoutView=listView&

# PART III

# CRACKS IN THE MONOLITH

## I 7

# "THE FISH IS ROTTING HEAD TO TOE"

For the most part, Poul Thorsen and NANEA were insulated from the outside world, and thus criticism. Protected by the CDC and all of its sub-agencies, the institutions in Denmark from SSI to Aarhus University, the mainstream press in the U.S. and U.K., and the stone-walling and delay tactics deployed by the U.S. federal government on FOIA requests, Poul Thorsen could do practically whatever he wanted to do. And he did—with zero oversight.

One time, a persistent father of an autistic son did get through to Dr. Thorsen. Smelling the rot of corruption that emanated from the Danish Studies, Brian Hooker, a professional engineer (PE) and PhD, could hang with anyone at the arrogant CDC or narcissist Dane Poul Thorsen and his posse any day of the year. Dr. Hooker was one of the relentless advocates for the truth of the vaccine cover-up at the CDC. From 2004 to 2005, the PE sent four FOIA requests to the CDC.

One request sought all written CDC correspondence regard-ing the Danish studies. The CDC sent these requests to the National Immunization Program, the National Center for Birth Defects and Developmental Disabilities, the National Center for Environmental Health and the Office of the Executive Secretariat for processing.

Ultimately the CDC withheld most of the responsive documents, claiming that they contained exempt information and opinions given by Danish researchers who were acting as "temporary consultants," authors of the study and researchers for the National Immunization Program.[168]

So the CDC's response to Dr. Hooker on Poul Thorsen and the NANEA team as being "temporary consultants" was a blatant lie. First, Dr. Poul Thorsen was a visiting foreigner scientist from Denmark, for which the CDC gave him a permanent CDC.gov email address and, so they thought, carte blanche access to CDC Federal Credit Union bank accounts. Not bad for a "temporary consultant." And then, year after year, CDC not only renewed its cooperative agreement with Thorsen for nine years running—had the "used car salesman" of a scientist not been caught forging CDC invoices—but they expanded the scope of that agreement. Nothing temporary about that.

From 1999 to 2000, spurred by the need of the CDC, Thorsen's research shifted from vaginas, preterm delivery, and underweight babies to cerebral palsy. That was part of the first CDC-NANEA cooperative agreement, by way of the Danish Medical Research Council and Ib Terp's signature. But politically savvy Terp never provided oversight from Copenhagen.

During the fallout from the Simpsonwood meeting of June 2000, with CDC Dr. Diane Simpson's ensuing, desperate search for data to manipulate the backtesting of a non-thimerosal nation, Thorsen's NANEA became fully engaged in adding autism and vaccine research to its areas of research in 2001. It would become his number one area of focus for the rest of the decade, since that is where the blood-sucking,

---

[168] *Dad Pushing Autism Link Can Get More from CDC,* by Erin Mcauley, Courthouse News Service (August 24, 2012) pg. 1.

money-orbiting opportunist saw the research funds pour in by the millions. All Thorsen had to do, as told by his bedside mole Dr. Diana Schendel, was to make sure his research group set out to disapprove any and all association between the mercury-based preservative and autism caused by vaccines.

By 2004, that scope would continue to expand further after the Danes were observed playing ball by CDC's executive branch: by running through many permutations—as many as needed—to warp analysis of data to make the conclusions hum and sing the CDC tune that "vaccines are safe." You can't question the science.

There was nothing temporary about that incestuous relationship between lovers Poul Thorsen and Diana Schendel, who mashed two of William Shakespeare's great plays, Romeo and Juliet and the very Danish Hamlet, into one twenty-first century amoral cesspool of likely scientific fraud, and at bare minimum scientific dishonesty.

The truth about the "dishonesty" came as a double gift in a pair of emails sent from Dr. Kreesten M. Madsen and Diana Schendel. On Friday morning of July 3, 2015, this surprised author finally—after six long weeks—received a response from Dr. Schendel, who wrote:

> Dear James Grundvig,
>
> In response to your email to me on May 29, 2015, I have no comment regarding Poul Thorsen. In the future, please direct your inquiries to Allan Flyvberg [sic], Dean, Faculty of Health Sciences, Aarhus University. For myself, I stand fully behind my research and my scientific integrity.
>
> Sincerely,
> Diana Schendel[169]

The "no comment" on her lover was expected. What was a surprise was her overreaction to the psychological pressure I applied in contacting

---

[169] Email from Diana Schendel to James Grundvig, July 3, 2015.

her. In telegraphing the scientist exactly what I was going to do with the book and sharing the sumptuous, titillating title, *Master Manipulator: The Explosive True Story of Fraud, Embezzlement, and Government Betrayal at the CDC*, she clearly felt an urge to protect her reputation and job at her new research gig at Aarhus University: the same university Poul Thorsen resigned from in 2009, and the same university where the new managing director had to "disown" Poul Thorsen—but his research?—in January 2010 from any and all future association. Schendel must have believed she insulated herself for being "transparent" for the first time in her career, because she unwittingly not only cc'd Dr. Allan Flyvbjerg, the Dean of the Faculty of Health Sciences, in her email, but she invited this author to contact him directly.

While most Americans enjoyed the Fourth of July weekend with the national holiday falling on a Saturday, I spent the weekend coming up with eleven pointed questions that I sent to Dr. Flyvbjerg the following Monday to answer on both Poul Thorsen and the so-called solid and untainted Danish studies.

I knew as a first generation Norwegian-American that Denmark, like the rest of Scandinavia, was on holiday for the month of July and that Allan Flyvbjerg's assistant would respond in mid August.

What drove Diana Schendel to seek what she believed was protection from her new higher ups at Aarhus University? Was it her guilt? The guilt of knowing the truth that she, along with her former CDC boss in Dr. Coleen Boyle and Poul Thorsen, knew about the "flattening" of data to show no association that autism, in fact, was on the decline in Demark after thimerosal was removed? Was it the tenuous feeling she had felt in 2009, being fingered as an accomplice in the Poul Thorsen financial crimes? Was it her fear of receiving her second letter of reprimand in six years from her employer, which could put her on probation again, and even fire her?

Whatever the reason, Dr. Schendel would survive the "meticulous" response Dr. Allan Flyvbjerg said would deliver. Unfortunately, he, like the CDC before him, whitewashed the answers.

In his three-page letter, dated August 20, 2015, Dr. Flyvbjerg answered my questions on behalf of Aarhus University.

1) Did Poul Thorsen break the Vancouver Protocol on scientific peer-reviewed papers by "doing little to no work" as Dr. Madsen had claimed in a telephone interview?

   "No, I have no reason to believe that the Vancouver Protocol was violated, all things considered."[170]

   **Comment:** That's because Dr. Flyvbjerg didn't bother to contact Dr. Madsen about the breach in scientific duty.

2) Is Madsen's supervisor still working at Aarhus University?

   Dr. Flyvbjerg: "Yes, the supervisor is still working at Aarhus University?"[171]

   **Comment:** This answer was expected, since Madsen's supervisor at the time was Jørn Olsen who is a professor at and head of the Danish Epidemiology Science Centre, AU, and since 2005, professor and chairman of the Deptartment of Epidemiology, UCLA School of Public Health. In other words, Dr. Olsen, who is a world-renown expert in the field of epidemiology, couldn't have that stainless reputation be soiled by the dirty dealings and multitude of crimes committed by Poul Thorsen.

By not contacting Dr. Madsen, who in 2015 worked as a medical doctor in the hospital district north of Copenhagen, Aarhus University by default continued to provide cover to its esteemed Dr. Jørn Olsen as opposed to finding the truth and rooting out all of the dishonest and illegal schemes perpetrated by Poul Thorsen. Olsen and Schendel both survived—at least for the near future—exhuming Thorsen's past, which easily could have tainted the former and

---

[170] "Concerning Your Letter Regarding Poul Thorsen," Dr. Allan Flyvbjerg, Aarhus University Health, letter on August 20, 2015.

[171] Ibid, pg. 2.

taken down the latter and should have been done in 2009. But CDC needed to keep Schendel and Thorsen quiet about what actually took place. The agency couldn't take the risk of firing Schendel or extraditing the fugitive Thorsen in real fear that they would talk, show where the skeletons resided in and which closets the bodies were buried.

Looking back, the U.S. Centers for Disease Control cemented the long-term, monolithic, permanent relationship not once, but twice. First in "2000 NANEA established a grant of $7.8 million from the American health institution Centers for Disease Control and Prevention (CDC). The grant was administered by Danish Agency for Science, Technology and Innovation (DASTI) under the direction of Poul Thorsen."

Then seven years later in "2007 the project was prolonged by a new grant from CDC of $8.2 million."[172]

With $16 million over sixteen years—had Thorsen not blown up the second long-term contract with the CDC—plus his three to four years of being a visiting scientist—had the Dane not been caught absconding—he would have had a relationship and partnership with science research projects that would have spanned twenty years. That is the same twenty years Diana Schendel fought to keep with the CDC in order to collect her full U.S. federal government pension. There was nothing "temporary" about twenty years, and there was never any "consulting" on the part of Poul Thorsen it was a one-way street that followed the whims and directions of certain individuals at the CDC on where, how, and when to play ball.

Brian Hooker, ever the don't-take-no-for-an-answer father and engineer when he is thrown a line of bullshit like "temporary consultant" moved outside the CDC and its email. Inadvertently, by giving Poul Thorsen a CDC email address. Well, Dr. Hooker went online

---

[172] *When the Agitator Came to the University,* by Sanne Maja Funch, www. Information.dk (March 13, 2010), pg. 8.

and found Poul's email address, the agency thought it would control the flow of information with the visiting scientist, but he had other ideas. Well, Dr. Hooker went online and found Poul's email address at Aarhus University. With that in hand, he sent the Danish scientist the following email exchange on November 24, 2004:

> I am and was Principal Investigator on CDC projects on Autism during those years. We are not trying to cover up any truth and we do not work on research more than 80 hours per week for nothing less but the truth or as close as we can get to it. We do not leave out any possible explanation including vaccinations and thimerosal in our work, anytime—we continue to question our findings andnew ones to come. The same do my colleagues at CDC and at SSI . . . —Poul.[173]

Brian Hooker, ever being respectful of Poul Thorsen and having no inkling that Dr. Thorsen had begun his new career of stealing money from the CDC, replied:

> Dr. Thorsen: Thank you for your response. Why did you choose not to disclose your affiliation with the CDC in the Madsen et al. 2003 publication?[174]

A bit ruffled by Dr. Hooker's pit bull–type persistence, Poul Thorsen rolled up his sleeves to blow off the American father of an autistic child, never once thinking that email along with the twenty-two counts of wire fraud and money laundering would come back to haunt him a decade later. Thorsen wrote:

---

[173] Email Nov. 24, 2004: NANEA Poul Thorsen to Dr. Brian Hooker.
[174] Email Nov. 24, 2004: NANEA Poul Thorsen to Dr. Brian Hooker.

Dear Dr. Hooker: The 2003 publication had nothing to do with CDC and was initiated without their involvement a lot earlier than my position as PI for autism projects and by other researchers in Denmark. All these questions have been answered by the corresponding author, previously. So please forward these question to the corresponding author on the 2003 publication in the future. Best Regards, Poul.[175]

From the numerous email communications from the CDC to Poul Thorsen, Diana Schendel, Kreesten Madsen, and so many more, the "2003 publication had nothing to do with CDC and was initiated without their involvement." is one of the great lies of this tragic, toxic saga, right next to Thorsen being labeled a "temporary consultant" by the CDC.

Just like Poul Thorsen falsely put his name down on at least two—if not several more—key research studies financed in part by CDC, the Dane appears to have been an amoral, ass-kissing, pathological liar.

The proof is in his own emails, credits where they shouldn't be, and a twenty-two count U.S. Department of Justice federal indictment.

But like all things that Poul Bak Thorsen underestimated over the past two decades, the U.S. might just extradite him one day with a new president in 2017.

---

[175] Ibid.

# 18

# POSTPARTUM NANEA

# (AKA, SHELL SHOCK AT NANEA)

In 2012, Dr. Brian Hooker took his CDC's FOIA requests, in which key parts had been redacted, making some of the information useless. Journalist Erin Mcauley wrote that U.S. Judge Amy Jackson's decision "could help Hooker, who has an autistic child pursuing a vaccine injury case before the U.S. Court of Federal Claims."[176]

Mcauley later writes in the same article:

> Jackson disagreed. "The court finds that the disclosure of a comment relating to Dr. Thorsen's personal life would not improve the public's understanding of how the government operates," she wrote. "There is no indication that CDC, the alleged victim, was complicit in the charged scheme to defraud the agency of over $1 million of research grant funds. So, the mere fact that Dr. Thorsen has been indicted does not transform his personal information into information about what the government 'is up to,' and it was properly redacted."

---

[176] *Dad Pushing Autism Link Can Get More from CDC*, by Erin Mcauley, Courthouse News Service (August 24, 2012) pg. 1.

On the contrary, Dr. Thorsen's "personal life" would indeed show exactly how the Teflon CDC had operated since being chosen in 1983 to lead the investigation (not) to find a link between the Agent Orange spraying and the tens of thousands of U.S. troops, their children and grandchildren, who were harmed by the biological warfare perpetrated by the U.S. Army, Air Force, Pentagon, and Presidents John F. Kennedy, Lyndon B. Johnson, and Richard Nixon on the battlefields of Vietnam from 1962–1971.[177]

Looking beyond Poul Thorsen's personal life and relationship with CDC Dr. Diana Schendel to see how he operated at NANEA is also very telling of how the CDC operated during the years: not once inspecting the books of NANEA over the first eight years of the cooperative agreements, lying to Brian Hooker about the Danish team being "temporary consultants," and never vetting Thorsen out as a competent scientist in the agency's desperate search to find the ideal nation host and existing pool of health and vaccine data to backtest in order to shield the U.S. immunization program.

The CDC Agent Orange debacle, namely the 101st Congressional 1990 Report on the agency and how it exonerated the U.S. government from all fault and liability from the decade-long dioxin spraying program, is exactly how the CDC has operated as a Teflon monolith for the past thirty-plus years. Perhaps U.S. Judge Jackson should read that brief so she wouldn't so systematically reject the emails on Poul Thorsen's between-the-sheets personal life with the Centers for Disease Control.

Personal life aside, Poul Thorsen was the P.T. Barnum of science research in Denmark. Beyond the Dane being a lousy professor, a poor teacher, an unskilled communicator to students, an incompetent scientist, and an alleged thief by the FBI and U.S. DOJ, Thorsen sucked at business, too.

---

[177] https://en.wikipedia.org/wiki/Operation_Ranch_Hand

He fully never appreciated how Steve Jobs and Steve Wozniak of Apple fame, Bill Gates and Paul Allen of Microsoft, or David Packard and William Redington Hewlett of Hewlett-Packard became successful. They were partners with opposite skillsets, who often disagreed in order to push their vision of change forward. In fact, neither Facebook's Mark Zuckerberg nor Amazon's Jeff Bezos started up all by themselves; they too had lesser founding partners who were sounding boards, helping to navigate unchartered technology and business course.

Not Poul Thorsen. He was a one-man show. The master manipulator knew little about how to build a research group. What he was good at was being an opportunist and leveraging his intended target. He was also a good schmoozer with scientists in need and had the one skill that mattered in his world: He could raise research money from an array of sources and keep it coming. But being the leader of North Atlantic Neuro-Epidemiology Alliances was a different matter.

To the CDC, Poul Thorsen projected the appearance that NANEA was larger than it actually was. Kreesten Madsen confirmed as much during our telephone interview on June 23, 2015, when he reacted to seeing the 2002 Web-scraped NANEA list of employees I emailed him. He said, "Yes, my name was on the NANEA website when it was up. But my name really shouldn't have been on it, since my pay came from Aarhus University. Many of the names on the page shouldn't have been on it either. Like me, they were based at the university in their departments. We didn't move off campus to NANEA's office."

Poul Thorsen's new office on the hill overlooked Aarhus Campus, which overlooked the city of Aarhus down in the valley. Perhaps that signified something to Thorsen, but it irritated many senior scientists who were more respected and experienced. But money could buy a lot, and Thorsen understood this. He was able to convince, perhaps in one meeting, that he wanted to move NANEA off campus however it was proposed to the university elders. In the back of his mind, he knew all too well that being off campus would enable him to build a kind of cult following, boast success, and keep the prying eyes of university heads from prying into his business. They obviously didn't object since Thorsen was the breadwinner with the CDC. And the money continued to flow into the coffers. Verily, Aarhus University received some of that payment, but Thorsen controlled the invoicing, the disbursing of payments, and keeping the books in order.

On the outside of NANEA's brick home, which had been converted to an office, Poul Thorsen had a metal, silver-plated name emblazoned on the wall that read, "NANEA - North Atlantic Neuro-Epidemiology Alliances." Instead of following the Danish culture of not bringing attention to oneself, Thorsen made sure that his neighbors, those who came to work at or visit NANEA's office, and those cars that drove by from Aarhus University's School of Journalism, up the hill from the off campus office, would see it.

But Thorsen took his ego of "I have arrived" many steps further than a platinum nameplate and a research group name that projected his team was much larger—an entire North Atlantic network—than it really was. Poul Thorsen's P.T. Barnum mindset often shined through. He also spent some of the autism research money from the CDC on NANEA "swag": little gifts, trinkets, and merchandise meant to brand NANEA as the great new company. There was the NANEA belt, the NANEA belt-buckle, and parties for all occasions, from winter to summer and all points in between, including holidays, birthdays, and more.[178]

In 2010, Danish freelance journalist Sanne Maja Funch was able to interview three former employees—or "temporary" contractors after the Danish tax authority stepped into the bankrupt research group in 2009. When I met Ms. Funch at a coffee shop in Copenhagen on Monday, June 1, 2015, she reviewed the Web-scraped NANEA list of

---

[178] *When the Agitator Came to the University,* by Sanne Maja Funch, www. Information.dk (March 13, 2010), pg. 4.

employees in 2002, shook her head, and said, "No, the three former NANEA employees I interviewed . . . are not on this list. They came to the research group later."

For her 3,300-plus-word article "When the Agitator Came to the University," Maja Funch said that she had to change the names of the three employees, who must have come to NANEA after 2005, to protect their identity from retaliation by either Poul Thorsen or Aarhus University. She was able to capture the demise of NANEA.

"I am ready to kill to my way,"[179] Poul Thorsen told his rapt employees.

> The sentence touches a nerve in Anja, when she listens to her chief talking about the ambitions that is the drive of his career. For one thing he is joking, but the joke and seriousness are as it is well-known complementary qualities, and Anja has seen and heard it all before. For many months she has worked at the research unit NANEA at the University of Aarhus. During that time she has experienced her chief, when he explains, that he is willing to sacrifice a friendship for a job, and that he does not care, whether there are more qualified candidates, if he himself is getting there first.
>
> Anja has seen what happens, when a new article is ready for publication, and the researchers are fighting about the order names in the byline of the article.[180]

Anja was not her real name. But the anonymous employee or independent contractor at the research group was one of a couple of dozen young, mid-level staff and interns who worked at the NANEA house on the hill. They were underpaid. When funds became thin and cash flow was a problem for NANEA, whether by Poul Thorsen's

---

[179]  Ibid, pg. 1.
[180]  Ibid.

alleged theft or mismanagement, the lowly staff suffered. Professional researchers like Kreesten Madsen, who had moved on from Thorsen, was never paid by NANEA, but by Aarhus University. Many of the top name scientists on NANEA's 2002 team in Ulrik Kesmodel, statisticians Anne V. Olsen and Heidi J. Larsson, consultants Ida Vogel Mogens Vestergaard, and project manager Puk Sandager[181] most likely were paid directly by AU. The midwives, nurses, and translators of NANEA were paid by the research group, but at either a low wage or as an independent contractor with few benefits.

On Anja's first day in meeting the researcher and data guru Poul Thorsen, she recalled him saying, "'You have to see opportunities!' It was Poul Thorsen's slogan, and I realize that he created an alternative research environment. It built on a principle of everybody being of equal value and everybody having something to offer."[182]

"'The entrepreneurial university,' he names the new era." Poul Thorsen said at an on-campus lecture that the "clever scientist is not only the one, who with hard work peels layer upon layer off human ignorance. Here the winner becomes the scientist who knows how to appear in a dynamic way and who is good at networking. It is him who is good at branding himself and his research and who is eager to be entrepreneurial and good at scraping money together."[183]

What Thorsen was driving at was the importance of the return on investment (ROI) in the world of research, or at least the appearance of that. Certainly the CDC thought they had stellar ROI with the Danish studies showing no link between MMR and thimerosal to vaccines. That allowed the vaccine-pharmaceutical-CDC monolith to operate unimpeded, business as usual. And it cost the CDC perhaps $25 million to build that shield of protection. Eleven million dollars

---

[181] http://web.archive.org/web/20021215062608/http:/www.nanea.dk/team/team_aarhus.html

[182] *When the Agitator Came to the University,* by Sanne Maja Funch, www.Information.dk (March 13, 2010), pg. 3.

[183] Ibid, pg. 5.

to Poul Thorsen, NANEA, and Denmark, plus another $14 million for travel, and CDC executive salaries over a number of years. Twenty-five million dollars to provide cover for billions of dollars of annual profits to the vaccine manufacturers deep into the twentieth century with many more vaccines coming online with the intent to be mandated by the United States federal and state governments.

No wonder Dr. Julie Gerberding left her colleagues Coleen Boyle, Bob Chen, Marshalyn Yeargin-Allsopp, Diana Schendel, Jose Cordero, William Thompson, Paul Stehr-Green, Roger Bernier, and so many others in the dust with her late 2008 announcement that she would resign as director of the CDC after ten short years with the agency to become the president of Merck's vaccine division; she knew where the real money was to be made.

At some point in 2006, Poul Thorsen must have heard a whisper from girlfriend Diana Schendel or he had a feeling that the CDC would most likely renew his contract. With the battle for MMR and thimerosal safety over, would the CDC need him or NANEA as much? Not knowing the answer, he planned for his future, just like Gerberding had deftly plotted the chess moves for her exit with the most golden of golden parachutes to join Merck in the most senior executive position. His plan was to up the frequency of stealing the CDC money by trying to cover his digital tracks; hers, to find a fall guy in case things went south and the public learned the truth about the years the CDC and NANEA went to bed to disprove any link between vaccines making money and the new childhood epidemic of autism, ADD, ADHD, and so many more disorders on and off the spectrum.

As the façade that had always been NANEA—neither an entrepreneurial research group nor the best dataminers of the Danish Health Registries—began to crack and crumble, Anja received a letter from SKAT, the Danish tax authority, which had been tipped off by a former employee, that she was "receiving public means that are unjustified." In fact, her salary, as it were, was against the law in Denmark. Thorsen had deftly used a "publicly financed tool to reduce unemployment."

More precisely, Anja got her supported salary and additional an additional amount that Poul Thorsen paid on top of that every month. "The end result for her is the correct salary for her full time employment. That is not legal."[184]

Like many other NANEA employees, Anja faced a heavy tax fine to SKAT. In essence, the guru screwed her to make more money for himself, verifying the statement by Kreesten Madsen that "Poul starved NANEA," financially speaking.

So to where did the $1 to $2 million or more disappear? The FBI knew the alleged fraud had begun at least fifteen months before Thorsen plunked down $33,000 for the Harley Fat Boy in Stone Mountain, Georgia.

In confronting the guru, Anja handed the letter to Thorsen showing the tax dated to the start of her employment at NANEA. "The tax case showed two things. One is the economy halted so much at NANEA that several employees are paid illegally. The other was that it is hopeless to speak to the boss about the problem. Poul Thorsen got 'woolly in his mouth,' when pressed for an answer, explained Toke. Everybody noticed that the man on the floor had absolutely no insight into the economy of NANEA."[185]

Instead of having answers for "Naneans"—the mascot name for his younger staff—such as Anja, Lise, and Toke, Poul Thorsen promised them, "new colleagues, who can start tomorrow, if only the Naneans work hard and help getting hold of financing." Not entirely buying it, he added with encouragement, "You must contribute to the pool for our common good. Then we will draw out the double amount next year. That is what you do in a family. You stretch out for one another."[186]

Soon the self-imposed exiled Poul Thorsen would abandon his Naneans in the house on the hill. He would let the coffers run dry in

---

[184]  Ibid, pg. 6.

[185]  Ibid, pg. 6.

[186]  Ibid, pg. 7.

2008 and let the university come in and investigate the research group the following year.

With no fear of consequence and a new CDC long-term coopera- tive agreement coming online soon, Poul Thorsen only "stretched" for himself, extending his hand out to take more money from his dying research group NANEA and the CDC.

# 19

# HIGH TIMES IN HOTLANTA

Addicted to cash and drunk with spending, Dr. Poul Thorsen took off on his red-and-chrome Harley Screamin' Eagle Fat Boy motorcycle. He zoomed around Echo Lake, a manmade reservoir three miles from North Druid Hills, then up main routes and down country roads searching DeKalb County, east of Atlanta, for a house to live in near the Centers for Disease Control headquarters. At forty-five years old, the Danish scientist had to be experiencing a sense of mid-life crisis mixed with an edginess of believing that he was so close as a scientist, on the verge of fame and glory and a major breakthrough.

Reality, of course, was quite different.

Some days Thorsen was on his own during the search for a house to live in; other days he took Diana Schendel with him on the Harley or in the Audi Quattro, which made him seem less of a risk taker when he met with the real estate agent, went to an open house, and met homeowners who were selling their houses.

For Diana Schendel, the house Poul Thorsen would purchase was an attempt at a solidifying their relationship, a chance to make their fondness for one another blossom and grow. After buying the Harley with one cool check at the end of May 2006, Thorsen would make his next withdrawal from the CDC by way of Aarhus University and NANEA to the amount of $52,892.25 on July 27, 2006.[187] The check was on a different CDC Federal Credit Union bank account that Thorsen opened. He would use it for a down payment on a four-bedroom house with small property—low maintenance—on Briarlake Road in Atlanta.[188]

The spacious European home, built in 1990, was "close to Emory, CDC, and major interstates. The home features hardwood floors on main level, gourmet kitchen with Corian countertops, cozy Living room with fireplace, office/library, master bedroom suite with fireplace, terrace level has apartment/in-law suite with full Kitchen and bath. Backyard has large new Deck for entertaining."[189]

On sale for less than $500,000, Poul Thorsen plunked down the 10 percent deposit and bought the house on August 11, 2006.[190] Just as he did with the CDC when he first came to "Hotlanta" to experience one of its brutally humid and hot oppressive summers in the late 1990s as a visiting scientist from Denmark, (and ingratiated himself with the agency executives while slipping into bed with Diana Schendel), he moved fast and deep. Thorsen wasted no time. In two and a half months, he bought himself a Harley and a dream house meant for raising a family.

By 2006, Diana Schendel was well over fifty years old and a highly improbable candidate to give birth as a first-time mother. Still, a family-oriented house with a coral exterior instead of a high-floor bachelor pad in a luxury condominium in Buckhead

---

[187] Case 1:11-cr-00194-UNA, Doc 1, Filed 4/13/11, "USA vs. Poul Thorsen" by U.S. District Attorney Sally Quillian Yates, pg. 6.

[188] Ibid, pg. 8.

[189] http://www.zillow.com/homedetails/2657-Briarlake-Rd-NE-Atlanta-GA-30345/14552734_zpid/

[190] http://www.trulia.com/homes/Georgia/Atlanta/sold/3126-2657-Briarlake-Rd-NE-Atlanta-GA-30345

must have reassured her about Poul's intentions. If Diana Schendel didn't know about her Danish boyfriend's alleged thieving ways by the time he closed on the house, dropping a cool $85,000 in cash in ten weeks without breaking a sweat, she either must have been naive, non-inquisitive, or a fool blinded by love and the salesman side of Thorsen.

But that would catch up to her, just as Thorsen's string of money withdrawals, wire transfers, and false invoices would eventually burn him. Money, when one is near a pile of it, can be such a blindspot for most people. It can change their behaviors, bringing out the beasts of envy, jealousy, and avarice in a heartbeat.

The house in Atlanta represented Poul Thorsen's ripcord to pull on when he would bail on NANEA and Denmark in late 2007 and live in the United States for good, and it gave Thorsen such a confidence boost. In his narcissistic eyes he looked in the mirror and nodded to himself that he had done a good job.

His payment for rewarding himself in solving the CDC's vaccine-autism crisis was to make a couple of more withdrawals in the first week of December, right after enjoying his first Thanksgiving dinner in his new home with Diana Schendel and friends. On Monday, December 4, and Tuesday, December, 5, 2006, Poul Thorsen would commit two of the first wire fraud counts in the amounts of $24,708 and $43,406, respectively, according to the federal indictment against him, "all in violation of Title 18/United States Code, Sections 1343 and 2."[191]

Why did Thorsen wire the oddball numbers of 708 and 406 as opposed to the rounded off amounts of 700 and 400? Who was he fooling? Or were those exact amounts? And were those wires sent back to bank accounts he controlled in Denmark?

---

[191] Case 1:11-cr-00194-UNA, Doc 1, Filed 4/13/11, "USA vs. Poul Thorsen" by U.S. District Attorney Sally Quillian Yates, pg. 5.

The U.S. Department of Justice officially stated "no comment" on the case since it is still officially under an open extradition proceeding of a wanted fugitive by the Office of Inspector General by the Department of Health & Human Services.

Once the $130,000+ had been successfully removed from CDC Federal Credit Union bank accounts he controlled in 2006—withdrawn in four large payments—he decided to up the game and make eight wire transfer and check payments, totaling more than $350,000. His most daring was on June 18, 2007, when he wire transferred $121,961, while his most unusual was on back-to-back days right before America's St. Patrick's Day celebration in March. On the 15th he wired $56,506 and the very next day he transferred almost an identical amount in $56,400.[192] Did he leave $106 behind to leave some money in the account for a reason?

As NANEA began to burn in 2007, Poul Thorsen would close on the next eight-year, $8.2 million cooperative agreement with the CDC. The Dane again went out and celebrated his good fortune and bought a 2008 Honda CR-V, EX-L, four-door SUV.[193] "The luxurious EXL trim gains dualzone automatic temperature control, premium audio and an eightway power driver's seat with power lumbar."[194]

Again, by year's end with no one asking him on either side of the Atlantic to look at NANEA's books, it only emboldened the thief to steal more from the money jar. So Poul Thorsen wasted no time in the New Year and made a wire transfer on January 16, 2008, in the amount $47,171. He would go on and make another nine counts of wire fraud and money laundering that year, totaling in excess of $330,000. The most activity came at the end when Poul Thorsen must

---

[192]  Ibid, pg. 5.

[193]  Ibid, pg. 8.

[194]  http://www.kbb.com/honda/cr-v/2008-honda-cr-v/

have known the party would soon be over. Probably aware that Dr. Julie Gerberding had secured her golden exit with Merck and would soon resign with a new U.S. president taking power in January 2009, which signaled a changing of the guard at the CDC, Thorsen was also keenly aware of the global economic meltdown in the financial markets in mid September. Five weeks later on October 29, 2008, he made three maneuvers with his CDC bank accounts. He wired two equal payments of $23,602—he had done the same exact thing earlier that June on a single day—and followed the coup-de-gras with a check transfer between two of his CDC bank accounts in the amount of $47,200, or just $4 shy of the earlier two wires combined.[195]

To the FBI and the U.S. DOJ, who made the indictment against public on April 13, 2011, Poul Thorsen allegedly absconded with more than $854,000, bought himself a beautiful four-bedroom home in a wealthy neighborhood of Atlanta, a kickass collector's edition Harley Davidson Fat Boy motorcycle, a luxury sports car in the Audi Quattro, and the Honda SUV.

Not a bad haul for a scientist who apparently did little to no research on several key studies he took credit for as coauthor against the Vancouver Protocol. For the unethical fugitive scientist, on some of the studies he had the CDC finance; if Thorsen is ever found guilty of all twenty-two counts in the U.S. DOJ indictment, then it becomes crystal clear he stole a lot more with the help of "known and unknown" conspirators in a ruse that ran for as long as five years or more.

Not only did Poul Thorsen waste money intended to go to autism and cerebral palsy research in order to stroke his ego with NANEA swag, the off-campus villa that doubled as an office in Aarhus, and throw feel-good winter, summer and holiday celebrations, but he also

---

[195] Case 1:11-cr-00194-UNA, Doc 1, Filed 4/13/11, "USA vs. Poul Thorsen" by U.S. District Attorney Sally Quillian Yates, pg. 5, 8.

screwed his Nanean staff by shorting them with the tax fraud scheme that burned them with the Danish tax authority.

But if people thought that opening internal probes in early 2009 would slow Poul Thorsen down, stop him from screwing people, or enriching himself in other ways, they would have been mistaken. Unlike when other Ponzi scheme architects are caught, Thorsen didn't make a mea culpa to the CDC, Aarhus University, Diana Schendel, his peers and researchers he worked with over the years, or those underpaid employees at NANEA. No, he looked for new ways to whore himself on unsuspecting people.

# 2 0

# FAST-ACTING DANE

If Poul Thorsen were a pill, he wouldn't be poison. He would be a human growth hormone that juices athletes beyond peak performance. He wasn't about to let Dr. Julie Gerberding's exit from the Centers of Disease Control or the internal probe by Aarhus University in early 2009 disrupt his plans or slow his dreams of success and his lust for power and attention.

Instead of cooperating with the investigation, he ignored AU's inquiries about what happened to $1 million of the two CDC cooperative agreements up to the end of 2008. Was it missing? Was it simply unaccounted for in sloppy bookkeeping? Did Poul Thorsen simply steal it? No, instead of holding up a white flag saying the jig was up, he continued to operate as if the probe didn't exist at all. He made himself totally unavailable and uncooperative.

At start of 2009, Aarhus University noticed something wasn't kosher about several invoices on CDC letterhead. They inquired about them with the CDC, which stated that the invoices didn't come from anyone at the agency. Puzzled, AU reached out to the chief accountant at the Odense University Hospital (OUH), since OUH was both a financial and science partner on many of the studies

Poul Thorsen and NANEA conducted over the years. In fact, their chief accountant Niels Henning Poulsen had been given authority to examine NANEA's books on behalf of the Danish Medical Research Council and then later DASTI when it took over. But Poulsen, like the CDC, never asked to examine NANEA's books. That was eight years with zero audits.

When Niels Poulsen finally began to do the forensics of OUH's books with respect to the NANEA project, he discovered the university hospital where he worked, and where many of the Thorsen studies were conducted, had its own shortfall in cash. *What the hell is going on?* he must have thought.

"Odense University Hospital (OUH) in Denmark lost 4.5 million Danish crowns (DKK) due to a Danish autism researcher, Poul Thorsen's US research grants,"[196] wrote Danish journalist Ulla Danielsen in her January 7, 2012, article.

As she followed the money trail in Denmark, where in January 2012, 5.76 DKK was equal to $1 USD,[197] poor Poulsen would end up taking the fall for Thorsen's alleged take crime while not once auditing NANEA since he was promoted to his position in 2006.

In a separate article by Danielsen, she wrote:

"Poulsen became chief accountant at OUH in October 2006 but lost his position in the autumn of 2011 only months before retirement. 'They wanted another chief accountant,' he says."[198]

OUH fired Niels Henning Poulsen because when an institution loses that much money, they need a fall guy to blame. No one on the

---

[196] https://nbjour.wordpress.com/2012/01/07/danish-odense-university-hospital-lost-four-five-million-dkk-by-poul-thorsens-research-grants/

[197] http://www.x-rates.com/average/?from=USD&to=DKK&amount=1&year=2012

[198] https://nbjour.wordpress.com/2012/02/15/researcher-not-university-hospital-accounted-to-us-cdc/

board of directors would fire themselves for the lack of audits when another man was chief accountant.

I tried reaching out to Niels Poulsen, another victim of Poul Thorsen's web of deceit, when I was in Denmark at the end of May in 2015. The the former chief accountant had opened his own private accounting firm in Odense city after his pension was slashed; he fell short of retirement from the university by a matter of months. But calls to his office arrived at a disconnected line. Other attempts by email failed. Poulsen must have earned enough, since being axed in 2011, to finally retire. With little to go on, OUH washed its hands of the lost grant money and considered it a "police matter."

Certainly, Poul Thorsen wasn't going to flame out Niels Poulsen's way, being fired short of retirement and taking the blame for perhaps the previous auditor's fault in not once looking at the books of the special CDC-NANEA project.

No, Thorsen was too clever and too full of pride and ego to face the so-called music to bow out gracefully, admitting to the many mistakes or criminal acts. In 2007, Poul through one of his CDC contacts ingratiated himself to join the American Psychiatric Association's (APA) Diagnostic and Statistical Manual of Mental Disorders, Fifth Edition (DSM-5) Task Force. He was directed to update the definition of what autism and its cousin Asperger's disorders were, among other disingenuous objectives.

From Thorsen's own "biographical sketch" when he was an adjunct professor at Drexel University in Philadelphia, he wrote:

> Dr. Poul Thorsen, MD, PhD has agreed that, from the time of approval through the publication of DSM-V, projected in 2012, (his/her) aggregate annual income derived from industry sources (excluding unrestricted research grants) will not exceed $10,000 in any calendar year.[199]

---

[199] http://www.rescuepost.com/files/thorsen---disclosure---1-22-10.pdf

For a man who pretended not to need more than "$10,000 a year" from being a part of the APA's high profile DSM-5 Task Force, Thorsen must have figured he could parlay that opportunity with new projects, more work, and networking with some of the world's top epidemiologists. In other words, he saw working on the task force not as an honor but as an opportunity to make more money. Throughout his cut-short twenty-year research career, despite the fact that he is still earning publishing credits into 2015, Thorsen always looked for the next opportunity, the next payday.

By 2008, after having supposedly worked on studies with scientists at Emory University, Thorsen again erected a buffer for the future in case all the money he withdrew from the CDC and NANEA somehow caught up to him.

From Emory University, Rollins School of Public Health, in its Spring-Summer 2008 newsletter, The Epi Vanguard, by Chairman Dr. Jack Mandel, in the "New Faces" section, it stated:

> Professor Poul Thorsen, MD, PhD, has joined the faculty of the Department of Epidemiology, Rollins School of Public Health, Emory University, from University of Aarhus, Denmark. Prof. Thorsen is not new to the department as he has been adjunct member of the faculty since 2003.
>
> Prof. Thorsen started his research career as medical doctoral student in 1987 on preterm birth and has been working within that research area since and he has published more than 30 peer-reviewed papers within that particular research field. Besides Preterm Birth Prof. Thorsen also study Autism, Cerebral Palsy, Down syndrome, Hearing loss and Developmental effects of fetal alcohol exposures.
>
> He founded the research group, North Atlantic Neuro-Epidemiology Alliances, University of Aarhus, Denmark, (NANEA, see www.nanea.dk), 8 years ago. The NANEA research group counts around 20 full time researchers and

similar numbers of part time researchers; all working within the research areas mentioned. The research approach includes exposures in pregnancy such as data from medical record data abstraction ... test for biomarkers in pregnancy ... test for maternal genetic factors.[200]

Emory's Chairman Dr. Mandel had no inkling in the spring of 2008 that the adjunct professor the Rollins School of Public Health hired in Poul Thorsen had been busy withdrawing and transferring cash payments across town from the CDC, pillaging the CDC Federal Credit Union bank accounts. Or that his new professor had bought an expensive Harley, a pair of pricey cars, and a spacious four-bedroom house all with U.S. taxpayer money, some of which might have funded a portion of the studies Thorsen's Danish team worked on with Emory University.

By taking this faculty position and having it announced in Emory University Rollins' newsletter, Poul Thorsen had no doubt lied on his work application with Emory, as well as not listed his plethora of conflicts of interest. And in doing so, he also broke Aarhus University rules, where he carried a second fulltime job as a professor back in Denmark.

Finally, Dr. Jack Mandel and those responsible for hiring Poul Thorsen were unaware that the dashing Dane was a "lousy" professor and had abandoned his own research group, which, if it did employ twenty people at that time as the newsletter stated, soon wouldn't employ any.

In the 2008 study "Autism Prevalence Trends Over Time in Denmark: Changes in Prevalence and Age at Diagnosis," by Erik T. Parner, PhD; Diana E. Schendel, PhD; and Poul Thorsen, PhD,

---

[200] http://www.sph.emory.edu/departments/epi/documents/Spring2008.pdf

published in journal *Arch Pediatrics Adolescence Medicine* in December 2008,[201] the author affiliations read as follows:

> Department of Biostatistics (Dr. Parner) and North Atlantic Neuro Epidemiology Alliances, Department of Epidemiology (Drs. Parner and Thorsen), Institute of Public Health, University of Aarhus, Aarhus, Denmark; and National Center on Birth Defects and Developmental Disabilities, Centers for Disease Control and Prevention (Dr. Schendel), and Department of Epidemiology, Rollins School of Public Health, Emory University (Dr. Thorsen), Atlanta, Georgia.[202]

So not only did Emory University announce Poul Thorsen's new full time position as adjunct professor in the Spring 2008 newsletter, but it was also published in the study, which listed NANEA and Aarhus University as well. They made Thorsen's dual work at both universities known to the public. Here, Thorsen didn't try to hide his new job or position as he knew it would be unlikely for Aarhus University to search for what he was doing in America. Like the absence of audits or request to inspect NANEA's books, Thorsen believed no one back at AU would ever find out, let alone see if he carried a second professorship position, which was against the century-old Danish university's rules.

Yet, there was a pragmatic side to Poul Thorsen. And that had to come from his family, his rural upbringing in the most rural part of Denmark—the farms at Sundsøre, today Skive, and Breum to the north. Poul's father, Niels Brandt Thorsen, was a farmer, who was born July 29, 1923,[203] but died at the early age of sixty-one years old

---

[201] *Autism Prevalence Trends Over Time in Denmark,* by Erik Parner, et al. www.archpediatrics.com, Dec. 2008;162(12):1150-1156

[202] Ibid.

[203] Gravestone for Grinderslev Church: http://www.danskkgindex.dk/grinderslev/grinderslev_visbilled.php?img=/grinderslev/pics/P1000065.jpg

on December 18, 1984. The death of Poul's father must have had a big impact on the twenty-three-year-old, who was either in or fresh out of college. Did the loss of his father negatively affect the young man? Did his father's death propel Poul to go into science and medicine? Or did the death of his father set the course for a young Thorsen to no longer fear or absolutely follow the orders of authoritative figures? And if the latter, was that the reason Poul Thorsen became an opportunist?

But perhaps because of his father's back-breaking, life-shortening livelihood of being a farmer—this author's father grew up on a farm in southeast Norway from 1913 until the start of World War II—in a long line of farmers, the young Thorsen decided to get educated and move into a higher profile avocation of science, medicine, and technology. By the 1990s, with his eyes set on America, the seduction of capitalism couldn't be far behind.

In an email from a Danish journalist to me on confirming Poul Thorsen's family tree, the reporter wrote: "Poul Bak Thorsen could be baptized in Grinderslev Kirke (Grinderslev Church – just outside Breum) – when I take a look at a database of the graveyard a lot of Thorsens seems to be buried there. It could indicate that the family farm is connected to that church."

Either way, Thorsen's upbringing of being pragmatic and thinking like a farmer in sowing the fields for next year's harvest came to bear with the recent discovery that he had secured a home in Stocksund, Sweden, a tony island that ensured privacy just northeast of Stockholm. The house address of Andistigen 180[204] showed his name in the Swedish yellow pages. A deeper search with a journalist friend of mine in Stockholm netted a 2009 real estate advertisement that publicly announced on September 1, 2009, that the house was sold to "Berit Agneta Blomgren."[205]

---

[204] http://personer.eniro.se/resultat/Poul+Thorsen/Stocksund
[205] "Center in Danderyd" Tuesday, September 1, 2009, on page 35.

A search of this Swedish woman's name showed her also own-
ing 181–182 Andistigen. That would make sense, if for her daughter
Agneta Blomgren lived at 180 Andistigen. In searching for her name
on LinkedIn, it would seem she is a "Volumetric Billing Specialist at
Hewlett-Packard" in Stockholm.

What seemed incredible, even ironic, was that Agneta Blomgren
and her mother Berit appeared in a E-Turbo-News article on tourists
visiting Wall Street during the fall 2008 crash:

> Outside the New York Stock Exchange hundreds of tourists
> joined police, TV crews, school children, hot dog vendors, and
> a whitebearded busker playing "Amazing Grace" on the flute.
>
> Swedish visitor Agneta Blomgren, 43, photographed her
> mother Berit outside the exchange. An electronic board dis-
> playing plunging share prices provided the backdrop.
>
> "We wanted to come and see it," Blomgren said. "The
> Americans aren't world leaders any more. It's time for a shift
> and this is the symptom of that. Power is shifting away perhaps
> to China."[206]

Being forty-three years old in 2008 means she was fifty years old
in 2015. Compared to Poul Thorsen's fifty-four years the red-haired
Agneta Blomgren could have been attractive to Thorsen.

With an internal investigation on the way at Aarhus University
in 2009, Poul Thorsen needed to be a few chess moves ahead of the
authorities, in case the probe got deeper and moved into criminality.
Ever the opportunist, the rogue Dane also needed a fall back position, a place outside of Denmark. With a retreat, or so-called place
to lay low, Thorsen sought and found that person in another woman,

---

[206] Tourists Flock to Witness Fall of Wall Street," by AFP, www.eturbonews.com,
October 12, 2008.

who fit the bill outside of Stockholm, Sweden. Were they more than just friends?

Thorsen's late father Niels would be proud of the farmer instincts in Poul of diversifying his exit strategies when his world would come crashing down.

Poul Thorsen didn't play by the Western rule of only one marriage at a time. He moved fast in America to secure as many mistresses (women and new jobs) as possible to satiate his desire for money, lust for fame and bedtime rendezvous, and to tap into the forever golden goose of opportunity.

"When the shit hits the fan, turn it on high," an old friend and anesthesiologist once told me.

That would become Thorsen's new motto.

He would put it to use sooner than he might have imagined.

# 21

# TRIPPING THE FAULT LINE

In mid-August 2014, a CDC whistleblower was outed at the worst possible time: the end of summer, when most people and the most powerful insiders in media are on vacation, schools are still closed, and when stories are meant to get buried, not exposed to the general public. Those who were guilty of that breach can learn and take a page out of TMZ Sports, which deftly broke the biggest sports story of 2014: the NFL's Ray Rice and Commissioner Roger Goodell debacle.

On Monday, September 8, 2014, the day after the first slate of NFL games were played that Sunday, TMZ Sports broke the story. The timing created a media buzz that spread around the country like an Internet virus. Timing was everything in blowing up the scandal that rocked the league and almost sacked the commissioner.

Long-time senior CDC Dr. William Thompson was that whistleblower. Outed prematurely after giving only four of perhaps what would have been a dozen recorded telephone interviews with Dr. Brian Hooker, Thompson had had his fill with the cabal of silence, the CDC's fabricated lies on vaccine safety in a tradeoff for the health of American babies, children, and teenagers. In seeing the skyrocketing rates of autism, which today exceed 1 in 68 babies born according to the CDC,[207] finally an agency insider, who worked with all the top executives over the years, had developed a conscience, a pang of guilt to which he could no longer hold back.

Dr. Bill Thompson, who lawyered up with the best whistleblowing law firm in the country, Morgan Verkamp LLC, had a lot more to divulge—at least for another six months. Because he had been outed with another three years left to work at the CDC to receive his government pension, the whistleblower clammed up.

In a press release statement issued by Morgens Verkamp, Dr. Thompson stated:

> My name is William Thompson. I am a Senior Scientist with the Centers for Disease Control and Prevention, where I have worked since 1998.
>
> I regret that my coauthors and I omitted statistically significant information in our 2004 article published in the journal *Pediatrics*. The omitted data suggested that African American males who received the MMR vaccine before age 36 months were at increased risk for autism. Decisions were made regarding which findings to report after the data were collected, and I believe that the final study protocol was not followed.[208]

Just like the Danish MMR and thimerosal studies had done, in manipulating the data to satisfy the main sponsor in the CDC, Bill Thompson admitted that he and others had deliberately omitted data on African-American children born in the Atlanta area. Had his discussions with Brian Hooker revolved only around that one study, then Poul Thorsen, Coleen Boyle, Diana Schendel, et al., the real master

---

[207] http://www.cdc.gov/ncbddd/autism/data.html

[208] http://www.morganverkamp.com/august-27-2014-press-release-statement-of-william-w-thompson-ph-d-regarding-the-2004-article-examining-the-possi-bility-of-a-relationship-between-mmr-vaccine-and-autism/

manipulators, might have been a moot point. But Dr. Thompson spoke at length about the corruption of science and manipulation of messaging inside the CDC. He blew the golden whistle.

On why thimerosal is still in U.S. vaccines, Bill Thompson had a very lucid, Occam's razor answer, saying:

> In the United States it is still in the vaccine for pregnant women. So, my theory on that, is the drug companies think that if it is in at least that one vaccine then no one could argue that it should be out of the other vaccines outside of the U.S. . . . So I don't know why they still give it to pregnant women, like that's the last person I would give mercury to.
>
> We know thimerosal causes tics. That's been demonstrated. That's been demonstrated in the big studies.[209]

So it appears that the FDA, CDC, NIH, and the Department of Health & Human Services are protecting the vaccine makers in a tradeoff of giving American babies, infants, and children tics—body tics, phonic tics, auditory tics, and fine-motor tics at bare minimum. But what if thimerosal was more harmful, even in minute amounts, than previously thought? What if thimerosal in concert with the three types of aluminum salts does a lot more damage to babies' immune systems, brains, neural networks, and lungs? Lungs in newborn babies are under development until the age of three years old—as told to me by my son's pediatrician, who warned in 2001, "No dunking in the pool for three years. The infant's lungs are still developing."

On Poul Thorsen and Diana Schendel, Dr. Bill Thompson had nothing nice to say. Besides Thompson going to town on the affair between the two research doctors, spending romantic summers in Denmark, taking strolls on the beach, he had this to say about Dr. Schendel. In

---

[209] *Vaccine Whistleblower: Exposing the Autism Research Fraud at the CDC,* by Kevin Barry, Transcript 1, May 8, 2014, pg. x.

2009, she had barely survived a CDC two-year letter of reprimand at the time Poul Thorsen had been exposed by the belated internal probes launched by CDC, OUH, and Aarhus University. Like the new managing director Jørgen Jørgensen, who had to come in and clean up the Poul Thorsen NANEA mess, Bill Thompson had to do the same with some of Schendel's half-baked studies.

> We have population controls of similar size (to Denmark) and we have disability controls of similar size. Now, this is the study I was brought in to clean up. Diana Schendel left town, left for Denmark, and I was brought in to clean it up. It's a big mess but regardless, there is now data available. Ya know, and there is going to be more data available. We're going to have 1,200 kids with autism as part of this study . . . with all of their medical records and all of their vaccine records abstracted. So, what's amazing, this is going to be shocking to you, it shocked the crap out of me. They have six different sites interviewing data and they all put in proposals to do studies.
>
> It's mind-boggling that it sat on one CD and actually the guy that had the one CD just came down with pancreatic cancer. Literally, that study data could have been gone for good. Anyways, so the name of the study is The Study to Explore Early Development. It's called SEED.[210]

Before she received the letter of reprimand as an accomplice to what Poul Thorsen had done, Diana Schendel was given the SEED program to lead, develop, and nurture. Bill Thompson must have rolled his eyes when he heard the news.

---

[210] *Vaccine Whistleblower: Exposing the Autism Research Fraud at the CDC*, by Kevin Barry, Transcript 2, May 24, 2014, pg. x.

Now there's one study that has been published from it, just describing the study and the sample. So, Diana Schendel is the first author. It's a 2012 paper, and you can just look it up. It might actually be on the website, I'm not sure. But, it's a Diana Schendel paper and it just pissed me off. I read it for the first time on Friday and she references two of her papers with Thorsen. I was just like, are you guys fucking insane![211]

They weren't insane. Diana Schendel, like her colleagues at the CDC past and present, learned from her boss, Coleen Boyle, over the years. If Congress never punished Boyle for her sins in the Agent Orange snow job, and the CDC didn't fire her but rather promoted her all the way up to being today the director of NCBDDD, the same position that Jose Cordero held at the start of the century, then it appears that by working at the CDC monolith one could only get in trouble if they didn't repeat the agency's line that all vaccines were safe. Anyone who challenged that proposition, like Bob Chen tried to do in a subtle sort of way, would get in trouble, sometimes serious trouble. Lying was fine. Fabricating data was fine. Cheating the system was fine. Screwing the American children was also fine. Transferring the costs of vaccine damage and all product liability to the parents of ASD children was very, very fine, stamped with approval by the U.S. federal government and Vaccine Court.

Diana Schendel was merely a cog in that loosely bolted vehicle, which had a Teflon exterior, projecting an aura of invincibility. But it had long run off the rails of science, ethics, and honesty. Dr. Thompson didn't want to stay on the ride any longer.

While Schendel worked behind the scenes to get the SEED project running as a template for other CDC autism projects, the pressure that Aarhus University's new managing director put on Poul Thorsen was too much to bear for the Dane by spring 2009.

---

[211] Ibid, pg. x.

With nowhere to hide in Denmark, Thorsen opted to run to America and other European nations that experienced an explosion of autism cases. The more sick and ailing the children there were, in population sizes magnitudes larger than Denmark, the busier he would become and the greater the opportunity—his favorite word. And because he could branch out, tap his connections, live off the stolen loot, and show his shape-shifting curriculum vitae, the better position he was in to land the next job or join a new project. And because he could work over the Internet, he didn't have to be in Denmark to tap into the Danish Health Registries of 200 databases, or design a study, or get his name as coauthor on some paper for which he would end up doing little to no work. He also had Diana Schendel, who was more than willing to do his bidding, to open doors for him, to connect him to the right people at the right universities on the right studies.

And Poul Thorsen had his Danish network to tap into as well.

Reading the NANEA writing on the wall that his days were numbered at Aarhus University, Poul Thorsen resigned from the university that made him, that gave him credibility, that educated him, that brought him notoriety within the small but significant world of epidemiology. And how would he show his gratitude for all those years of mentoring, the opportunity to be a professor—even as lousy teacher in the opinion of one former student—office space, and investment? (Yes, investment.) Would he pay the goodwill back to the university? No, apparently not. Instead, he would misrepresent an ongoing association with AU, bury the internal probes of his research group, and lie about his affiliations without blinking.

So proud is Emory University today for not fully vetting Poul Thorsen, when a phone call or email to Aarhus University's epidemiology department could have warned them about the marauding Dane.

Showing neither shame nor remorse, Poul Thorsen resigned from Aarhus University as a professor and research scientist—before incoming Managing Director Jørgen Jørgensen could swing the axe down on him and decapitate his career in a public spectacle worthy of a gathering before an old French guillotine.

Thorsen had tripped his own faultline with a seismic wave destined to follow. There was no way around that, nowhere for him to ultimately end up. Not with the Navy SEAL double tap of Aarhus University disowning him and the U.S. Dept. of Justice well on the road to indicting him.

On January 22, 2010, in an extremely rare public statement from Jørgen Jørgensen disavowing the university of any and all associations with the incompetent scientist, he wrote:

In March 2009, Dr. Thorsen resigned his faculty position at Aarhus University. In the meantime, it has come to the attention of Aarhus University that Dr. Thomsen [sic] has continued to act in such a manner as to create the impression that he still retains a connection to Aarhus University after the termination of his employment by the university. Furthermore, it has come to the attention of Aarhus University that Dr. Poul Thorsen has held full-time positions at both  Emory University and Aarhus University, simultaneously. Dr. Thorsen's double Full-time employment was unauthorized by Aarhus University, and he engaged in this employment situation despite the express prohibition of Aarhus University.[212]

Like the South Korean *Sewol* ferry captain, who abandoned ship leaving more than 300 people—most of them children and teenage students—to drown and die, Poul Thorsen turned in his resignation letter and bolted from Aarhus to America.

He fled from his dream research startup NANEA in that brick house on the hill above the campus. In Thorsen's eyes and to that of his

---

[212] Aarhus University Statement, from Jørgen Jørgensen, January 22, 2010, pg. 2.

jealous rivals—the more experienced scientists at Aarhus University—
NANEA's house looked down on the campus, as if it were superior to
the century-old university. What it exposed instead was Poul Thorsen's
inferiority complex, since he was not as talented a doctor and research
scientist as his peers. Worse, he left his former employees holding the
bag of debris of his wreckage. He abandoned them. He left many of
the young staff holding the tax scheme issue, too. He left them hanging in the wind to sort out their own affairs, as he flew back to Atlanta
to live large in the spacious house near beautiful Echo Lake, to search
for new work and make even more money. At each stop along the way,
he claimed to still work as a top research scientist at Aarhus University,
never once letting his new prospective employer know that he had
resigned, that there was an ongoing investigation into millions of CDC
dollars, or that he screwed his own underpaid employees, kids in their
twenties who were simply looking to start or build their early careers.

Thorsen left them in an empty house with boxes strewn, papers
scattered, and NANEA swag sitting on desktops and shelves. While
AU investigators pored over the files and details of the NANEA shipwreck, the Naneans either became unemployed or were folded into
the university. Kreesten Madsen, wanting no association with Poul
Thorsen, had bolted Aarhus before Thorsen left, probably sensing the
collapse of NANEA long before anyone else did.

In examining the Web-scraped 2002 NANEA employees list by
tracking down all two dozen of them and what they are doing today,
reviewing their LinkedIn profiles, and reading some of their online
resumes, not a single one had put NANEA as a place of employment
in their past. And remember, Mayor Ib Terp just shook his head refus-
ing to even admit that he knew Poul Thorsen, let alone was his keeper
in the early years of NANEA. Talk about radioactive.

Either the former employees put Aarhus University research in lieu
of NANEA on their resumes, or they simply left those years off. It was
that simple. Erase, forget, and move on, as if they had been a victim of
white-collar crime or emotional rape.

It was remarkable to see, really. To see how many, at one time, had bought into the guru of Danish Health Registries and his vision, dream and cult, and had since removed the stain and foul odor of Thorsen's persona or the association with the fugitive from the U.S. riding the Harley Fat Boy. Since they left, no one really wanted to talk about it. Kreesten Madsen became the only one, as he felt used by Thorsen when the founder of NANEA falsely put his name on the studies that Dr. Madsen had carried out.

On June 2, 2015, my last day in Denmark before returning to the U.S., I received Dr. Ida Vogel's reply to my email. Back in the Nanean day, Dr. Vogel was a "consultant" to NANEA; today she works at Aarhus University Hospital. She wrote:

> Dear James.
>
> I have done a substantial amount of research with Poul on preterm delivery some years back. I am sure of the high quality of all the studies I have been involved with. As for the financial case between Poul and the CDC I have no relevant information—I was never involved in the financial part of running NANEA. Regarding the more personal sides of the working relationship with Poul I am not interested in participating. I continue my hope that Poul is innocent until the Danish or the US system determines otherwise.[213]

On Friday on the eve of U.S. Independence Day, Diana Schendel sent an email to me. She must have thought long and hard about my trying to interview her after I came to Aarhus University, went to the third floor of the epidemiology department, and slid my business card under her office door.

I missed bumping into her by a few minutes.

---

[213] Email June 2, 2015: Dr. Ida Vogel, Aarhus University Hospital, to James O. Grundvig.

By cc'ing the Dean of Health at AU, Allan Flyvbjerg, Schendel believed she was covering her professional tail since she had become a full-time faculty member at Aarhus University in 2014. But in cc'ing the Dean of Health, she had unwittingly given this author a contact very high up in the university hierarchy to bring my questions to bear on what exactly took place at AU some dozen years ago.

Dean Flyvbjerg, in turn, expecting to see only a few softball questions on Poul Thorsen, must have been taken aback by the depth and breadth of the eleven questions I asked, the backup I provided, including CDC emails and a copy of Jose Cordero's infamous letter, and the fact that I had spoken—the first one to crack the inner circle of Thorsen—to Kreesten Madsen.

One of the eleven questions I asked centered on Diana Schendel's involvement in the CDC's decision to omit the 2001 data from the thimerosal study. The answer she will provide to Aarhus University might define how good her "integrity" of science is.

For Poul Thorsen, he was more than a pariah. He was a scam artist only out for himself. But like the U.S. federal indictment stated, he had a lot of help along the way.

Free after submitting his March 2009 resignation letter, however temporarily, he carried on misusing AU's name and his association to drum up new work.

Thorsen plunged headlong into finding the next project, like a drug user bent on trying to achieve the next high.

## 22

# OVERCOOKING THE DANISH

Sitting in the backyard deck of his house in Atlanta, under a starlit night, Poul Thorsen ran a cold bottle of beer over his forehead to wipe the sweat off. Hot and humid even after the sun set over Echo Lake, Thorsen congratulated himself on doing a great job in preempting any fallout from Aarhus University's new administration coming into office on Wednesday, April 1, 2009.

He hoisted that European beer and said "Skoal!" to the god of fate, whoever might be covering his ass when he had bailed on Aarhus and his Naneans.

By resigning, Thorsen believed that AU wouldn't come out and broadcast his departure. No one outside the city of Aarhus knew he had left. It was a preemptive move he made from being fired. That bought him time and quelled any scandal or bad press, at least for the near term. And it still allowed him to network with other people, scientists, and acquaintances and tell them all that he was still deeply involved with the epidemiological research being done at Aarhus University.

Sitting back and enjoying the beer, Thorsen thought about his good (enough) friend Dr. Alvaro Ramirez. He thought about the

November 2007 European Autism Information System (EAIS) Conference, where Dr. Ramirez presented an update on the EAIS project, which had drawn to a close in June 2008, after a thirty-month pilot study that Thorsen was involved in, in which Ramirez had dedicated three slides in the twenty-five-slide deck to Thorsen's participation in the project.

Partially funded by the European Commission's Programme of Community Action in the Field of Public Health (2003–2008), Thorsen recalled how scientists in attendance were trying to get a handle on the autism prevalence in Europe and how to measure it. Was it the Centers for Medicare & Medicaid Services' ICD10? Or the APA's 1994 DSM-IV? Or the French method? No one knew. Not even in 2009, two years later.

Dr. Ramirez clicked on slide fifteen, "Database for ASD Surveillance," and explained Poul Thorsen's three key contributions to the pilot study:

1) Working with Information Systems;
2) Instruction Manual;
3) Online Database.[214]

With his name reading on the slide—"Poul Thorsen, MD, PhD, NANEA, University of Aarhus, Denmark"[215]—Alvaro spoke about the technology of databases as if Poul Thorsen was an expert in big data such as Hadoop, Oracle SQL, and IBM. When Dr. Ramirez clicked to the datamining slide of Denmark's Health Registries, he knew Thorsen felt at home since the Dane was the one with the help of the CDC to leverage and backtest data across a spectrum of

---

[214] Dr. Alvaro Ramirez Deck: *European Autism Information System,* EAIS-Project Alvaro Ramirez (looking a lot like Martin Knapp), slides 15-17.
[215] Ibid.

diseases, disorders, and human conditions. But Poul understood as much about technology as he did about running a university research group or launching a business startup. He was vitamin "T" deficient, as in clueless about Technology.

That day, Dr. Ramirez clicked the next slide and felt he hit Poul's sweet research spot in "Population-based studies," listing eight European countries with the question "Where are the Pilot Studies?" The eight countries were "Spain, Italy, Portugal, Poland, Ireland, Luxembourg, Czech Republic, and Malta."

Understanding that the EAIS project had closed and achieved many of its goals, Thorsen focused on the brainchild project that he and Diana Schendel had cooked up in 2008. The European Network of Surveillance for Autism and Cerebral Palsy (ENSACP) was partially financed by the European Executive Agency for Health and Consumers.

Yet Dr. Alvaro Ramirez was frustrated with the postponement of the project's kickoff meeting date, delayed by several months.

Sweating, swigging beers, watching fireflies blink on and off in the night, Thorsen knew he couldn't postpone that meeting again, which was to be held June 6–7, 2009, in Wolfheze, Netherlands, a quaint Dutch village an hour's drive southeast of Amsterdam.

There he, Dr. Alvaro Ramirez, and Diana Schendel via Skype, along with nine other scientists, met at the summit to develop the ENSACP surveillance network for Europe.

Had Poul Thorsen taken out a pen that night and doodled a napkin sketch on what the future of autism incidence would look like in Europe, it might look very much like what a slide from 2010 EAPHA deck, "The Strategic Planning for Autism in Europe: Past, Present and Perspectives."

- From CDC's 2010 reported 1:110 Children at 8 years old.
- European Population 2010 = 500 million.
- European Estimated ASD Rate = 5 million.

- Affected Population 5% = 25 million population the size of Belgium and The Netherlands.
- Social Mortality Rate Indicator.[216]


But Thorsen wasn't interested in any such calculation or what it meant for the future of Europe. He knew the "affected population" meant the parents and siblings of those children, and how their lives would change, too. Either way it was a big fat number. He realized it would probably become worse by 2025 or 2030. Much worse.

At the meeting, Thorsen would tap Dr. Alvaro Ramirez to get himself more involved in the Irish Autism Action network, backed by the University of Cork College in Cork, Ireland. With not as many irons in the fire as he would have liked in Europe, Thorsen needed to network at the upcoming weekend conference. He needed to do it in a subtle way to secure some new post in the United States without showing how desperate he was, since he was cutoff from the CDC-AU-OUH cash cow.

At the Dutch hotel, where the ENSACP Conference was held, Poul Thorsen gave a presentation on "Biomarker Review for Cerebral Palsy." He opened by emphasizing the importance of coming up with a clear definition of the term "biomarker" in the context of their project.

"Physiological or pathophysiological biochemical or biomolecular alteration at the organ, tissue, cell, or sub-cellular level in response to an exposure that is measurable in biological samples and becomes the signature of the onset of disease, underlying disease process or phenotypic outcome,"[217] Dr. Thorsen said in an erudite-sounding, clumsy and roundabout way. His choice of using jargon-loaded language didn't help his cause to define "clearly" what the

[216] Autism Dublin 2010 - *European Autism Action 2020: A Strategic Health Care Plan,* slide 10.

[217] ENSACP Minutes of the Meeting, Transcript, June 6-7, 2009, pg. 4. http://www.docstoc.com/docs/84008671/ENSACP-Minutes-from-Wolfheze-meeting-June

term biomarker meant. But then, teaching or articulating scientific concepts in plain language with storytelling flair wasn't Thorsen's strong suit.

The Danish brainchild behind ENSACP addressed his fellow scientists in attendance by saying that his research on cerebral palsy biomarkers was "inconclusive" and needed more work, despite the fact that he had studied, researched, and written about the childhood disease for a decade. Maybe that was Thorsen's trick. Maybe that was how he sustained work and put his names on all of those studies, even though he did "little to no work" on some of them, according to principal investigator Kreesten Madsen's account. Thorsen milked the system of money by perpetually keeping the scientific conclusions open. Incompetent scientist, maybe. Good milkman, no doubt. No wonder he switched to the always open, non-conclusive ailments of autism and CP biomarkers. He, like the CDC who influenced the visiting foreign scientist, figured those afflictions would never get solved in his lifetime. Pure genius. Silicon Valley venture capitalists call that business model "reoccurring revenue."

It was all good, except for his greed and quest for vainglory.

At the end of his presentation, Dr. Poul Thorsen admitted further research was needed. Indeed. That meant more research dollars had to be raised to conduct the open-ended investigation. Of course, it was all about the money. Thorsen did commit to the group that he would complete the CP biomarkers report by the last week of September 2009.

"The final result will be presented at the October meeting. The delay of this deliverable will be considered in the amendment of the project,"[218] Thorsen told his colleagues.

To his credit, Dr. Alvaro Ramirez didn't buy Thorsen's excuse or let him off the hook with respect to the delayed report. Dr. Ramirez summed up the meeting with a series of questions on why Thorsen:

---

[218] Ibid.

- Delayed the kickoff meeting.
- Needed extra time to finalize the deliverables committed for WP4 and WP5.
- Needed more time for the description of the databases.
- Needed more time for the study proposals of the Work Packages (WP).
- Clarity on the amendment required to the project agreement with EAHC.[219]

For the first time since he met Poul Thorsen back at the EAIS project in 2006 in Ireland, Alvaro had his doubts about the Dane research scientist. Was he spread too thin? Did he stretch himself too far across continents?

What Alvaro Ramirez didn't know was the dark side of Poul Thorsen, the thief who stole from the CDC, OUH, and Aarhus University, leaving a debris field behind him of real victims. Ramirez also didn't know about Thorsen's hasty exit from AU, or his resignation letter, or the fact that he was Diana Schendel's long-time lover.

In reaching out to Alvaro Ramirez for an interview through several channels, he chose not to talk about defunct ENSACP or the half-baked EAIS project, or Thorsen's work at Irish Autism Action in conjunction with the University of Cork College.

The next ENSACP meeting was scheduled for October 15-16, 2009, to be held in beautiful Killaloe, Ireland. But like the original kickoff meeting, it would end up being cancelled, too, since Poul Thorsen would spend more time looking over his shoulder, searching for work, networking, and talking about how important his research was than working on the CP biomarkers report. Again, he failed to deliver the deliverables he promised at the ENSACP group of highly distinguished professionals.

---

[219] Ibid.

Would Thorsen and Schendel's ENSACP project survive in 2010?

By autumn 2009, Poul Thorsen felt the pressure from the lack of cash flow, from inquiries by Aarhus University and OUH's chief accountant Niels Henning Poulsen, and from rumors he heard from within the CDC that he had been deliberately thrown under the bus by one of the executives there. But who did that? Was it Coleen Boyle? Marshalyn Yeargin-Allsopp? Paul Stehr-Green? Bob Chen, who never really liked Poul Thorsen? Or someone else in power?

If someone at the CDC made Thorsen the fall guy in case the manipulation of data on those many faux studies was ever exposed, they could just point the finger and blame the Dane. If only he hadn't stuffed his hand in the money jar, bought the limited edition Harley, Audi Quattro, Honda SUV, half-million dollar home in a tony suburb of Atlanta, flew first class, took limousines here and there as if he was a rock star, wine and dined and bedded Diana Schendel, stuffed money meant for autism and vaccine safety research away in some likely off-shore bank account—then he could have defended himself. But he was trapped no matter who dropped the flag on him.

In postponing the ENSACP meeting, Thorsen turned his sights on securing another professor post. Turned down by John Hopkins University for such a role according to an anonymous source—perhaps the medical school learned he was a below average teacher—Poul Thorsen did manage to land a similar job 100 miles north of Baltimore in Philadelphia at Drexel University.

The post Dr. Thorsen would land was in the Neurodevelopmental Disorders Work Group as an adjunct associate professor in the Department of Epidemiology and Biostatistics, School of Public Health at Drexel. Certainly, he used his Emory University professor position, his work as a member of APA's DSM-5 Work Group, and his contacts at the CDC—most likely Schendel since he wasn't sure who dropped the money-marker on him in the agency about forging fake invoices.

Located in the Bellet Building at 1505 Race Street, Poul Thorsen worked at the medical school, which was located in Center City, some twenty blocks east from where Drexel University's main campus was located next to the University of Pennsylvania in West Philadelphia. His initial job, which began in December 2009, was a professor for a class of one, as in one PhD candidate student.

If his one PhD student didn't show up, Dr. Thorsen wouldn't have much to do in the way of teaching. Maybe that was a good thing. But after stealing money from the CDC and then watching the cash spigot get shutoff, the real world experience of having to go find work had to get to him.

Shutout from his homeland of Denmark to a great degree, he now found himself with few institutional jobs, few projects, and few studies. The one Drexel student would hold his interest to some degree, but it wouldn't slake his thirst for more robust and meaningful work, such as participating in studies. But he needed the money and the ability to tell people that he landed the new gig at Drexel University as bait to fish for a bigger, better-paying job or project.

In an email response to my inquiry on Thorsen's short-term work at Drexel:

James,

Poul Thorsen was an adjunct at Drexel's School of Public Health from Dec. 11 (2009) until he resigned his appointment with the School of Public Health on March 9, 2010. During that time, his role was limited to serving as a member of the thesis committee of one doctoral student.[220]

—Niki Gianakaris, M.A.,
Director, Media Relations,
University Communications at Drexel University

---

[220] Email April 15, 2015: Drexel University Niki Gianakaris to James O. Grundvig.

Poul Thorsen missed Denmark. He missed the camaraderie of working with like-minded scientists. He missed the rush of withdrawing large sums of money from one of his five CDC Federal Credit Union bank accounts. He missed his little Naneans he screwed over. He missed being with Diana Schendel the most. Just the sound of her husky voice turned him on, as did the memory of her soft, delicate fingers running through his hair.

Thorsen would fly to Atlanta for the holidays. He would ride his motorcycle around, enjoy a sightseeing trip with Schendel in his Honda SUV, spend quality time with her, and hope the new year of 2010 would bring something new, something special, something fulfilling.

## 2 3

# THE GREAT UNRAVEL

At the start of the New Year in the new decade, Poul Thorsen's dream of a fresh start got intercepted like a heat-seeking missile. He was shot out of the sky on January 22, 2010, by two pieces of paper almost identical in weight and size to what he sent to Aarhus University as forged instruments, the fake invoices on CDC letterhead.

That cold January day, Poul Thorsen didn't see the delayed counterpunch coming. Had he, he might have ducked. Instead, he took the blow square in the jaw. It knocked him back several steps. Dazed him. Stunned him. He waltzed about trying to find the corner seat or ropes of the ring to hang on; he clutched nothing but air.

Jørgen Jørgensen had thrown the hook that Thorsen never saw coming. In his highly unusual, terse, direct statement on the behalf of Aarhus University, the new managing director had thrown Poul Thorsen not only under the bus, but also pushed him and that bus off the cliff. Flailing about in reaction to AU's January 22nd press release, everyone from California and Atlanta to Ireland and Denmark knew the dashing Dane was in deep trouble. And if he had lied to certain people for the past eight months about still being employed at Aarhus University, then he was finally exposed as a fraud and a liar. The small world of epidemiology that Poul had trolled since resigning from the university a year before suddenly got smaller, and people would learn within a week or two that the Poul Thorsen scandal was real.

On the same day as the statement was released by AU, Dr. Thorsen had to revise his "bio sketch" on the APA's DSM-5 member Disclosure Report. Why? In Jørgensen's statement, he called out Poul Thorsen breaking university policy for working as a professor at two universities at the same time:

"Furthermore, it has come to the attention of Aarhus University that Dr. Poul Thorsen has held full-time positions at both Emory University and Aarhus University simultaneously. Dr. Thorsen's double Full-time employment was unauthorized by Aarhus University, and he engaged in this employment situation despite the express prohibition of Aarhus University."[221]

Dr. Thorsen must have peed in his pants when he got wind of the statement outing him as a fraud and schemer while under a police investigation. Cornered, he instantly had to update his January 12th DSM-5 Disclosure Report that read:

**Name:** Poul Thorsen, MD
**Job Title:** Professor
**Address:** Rollins School of Public Health
              Emory University
              1518 Clifton Rd, Room 256
              Atlanta, GA 30322
**Role:** Member
**Date:** 1/12/2010
**Work Group:** Neurodevelopment[222]

---

[221] Jørgen Jørgensen Statement on "Dr. Poul Thorsen," at Aarhus University (Jan. 22, 2010), pg. 2.

[222] *A new paradigm for a post-imperial world: Poul Thorsen's Mutating Resume*, by Dan Olmsted & Mark Blaxill, Age of Autism (April 5, 2010).

In taking advantage of Denmark being six hours ahead of the east coast of the United States, Thorsen changed his DSM-5 Disclosure Report to read:

**Name:** Poul Thorsen, MD
**Job Title:** Adjunct Associate Professor
**Address:** [Didn't name Drexel University here]
      1505 Race Street,
      Bellet Building, 11th Floor
      Philadelphia PA 19102-1192
**Role:** Member
**Date:** 1/22/2010
**Work Group:** Neurodevelopment[223]

Dr. Thorsen wrongly believed that making such a subtle change as removing the appearance of a "double" professorship at Emory University would somehow stave off the inevitable demise of his epidemiology career. It did not.

Anyone with an iPad or mobile phone could have searched Poul Thorsen's name in the vast network of the Internet and that statement would surface in the top five articles about him that winter. In essence, he was screwed by a piece of paper.

It didn't take long for other organizations, universities, and projects in his field to catch on that his name was mud. Soon those entities and associations he had been involved with would begin to click off the lights, like tripping circuit breakers in a house, turning one room after the other dark. It was akin to how the regressive form of autism works in shutting down the milestones that normal infants make in speech, eye contact, and fine motor skills over their first two years of life, in which the dreaded disorder begins tripping the circuit breakers inside the child's brain and body, in terms of functionality.

---

[223] Ibid.

Before the shit hit the fan, Poul Thorsen desperately needed his brainchild ENSACP's second meeting to work. The new date was set for February 20-21 and would take place at the Sheraton Hotel, Heathrow Airport in London, UK.

The lineup was a bit different than the original kickoff meeting for ENSACP in the Netherlands back in June 2009. For one, CDC Diana Schendel wasn't involved. No Skype from Atlanta. Was that due to Poul Thorsen protecting her association with him? Or more likely, was it due to her two-year probationary letter of reprimand as being a suspected conspirator with Poul Thorsen?

Dr. Alvaro Ramirez opened by emphasizing "that all the work produced on the ENSACP project must add up to an excellent final result."[224] He then apologized for Guy Dargent, Rotger Jan van Gaag, and Simon Baron-Cohen not being able to attend the meeting—even though Baron-Cohen lived and worked in London.

Perhaps, he and the others got wind of the statement from Aarhus University exposing the scientific fraud Poul Thorsen committed.

After that, Alvaro introduced Kevin Whalen, CEO of Irish Autism Action, which since its inception in 2001 had launched thirteen special education schools for autistic children. He turned to business and began by commending Poul Thorsen on the quality of work as "technical coordinator of the three main actions for the final phase of the project"[225] by the partners at their first technical meeting in Wolfheze, Netherlands.

Over the two-day meeting, Poul Thorsen explained that the three papers would be submitted to *Acta Obstetricia at Gynecologica* Scandinavian journal. He discussed money, in which the main author would receive around $2,000 when the article was published.[226] Of

---

[224] http://www.docstoc.com/docs/74849133/london_minutes

[225] Ibid.

[226] Ibid.

course he talked about money. He needed some. And that motivated him.

The carrot for Thorsen was money, to get paid for being an author on a study. To that end, Dr. Alvaro Ramirez discussed the "appropriate mechanism to proceed in this case, as it is important to maintain full transparency in all financial matters."[227] That line must have punched Poul Thorsen in the gut. The dirty Dane was anything but transparent. He operated in the shadows but claimed to work in the light of day.

Later on in the meeting, Poul discussed the Danish data system and BioBank, which was based at Statens Serum Institut. He told his peers that twelve students had been trained on the Health Registries and that "through a computer to a server" they could "extract the data." He said the cloud-based system was easy to use and up to date.[228]

What Thorsen didn't say at the meeting was how he screwed twelve similar students at NANEA with their wages and taxes and how he left them high and dry to fend for themselves with the Danish tax authority. Instead of sharing such a result of his awful behavior and treatment, he went on to talk about the "importance of having a description of the group of risk factors" associated with ASD.[229]

He then talked about the importance of data indexing, as if he were a coder, computer programmer, or database architect. He was none of them. Perhaps that was the way Poul operated: Size up the audience, figure who they are not, and talk about that "not" as if he was an expert. That method could have been risky from time to time, as he might come across a professional in finance who might code on the side, but that was a small risk he was willing to take, knowing that the chances of that happening in a small meeting of a dozen people, most of whom were scientists he knew.

---

[227] Ibid.

[228] Ibid.

[229] Ibid.

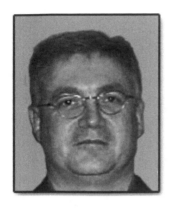

Poul Thorsen

Then Poul dropped the subtle hint. He reminded all present that he "would be working full-time" (for a change) on ENSACP project and that the final version of deliverables items Nos. 6, 7 & 8 would be finished by March 31, 2010.[230]

But as good as that promise sounded, after Alvaro Ramirez had commended Thorsen on the work he had done since the 2009 kickoff meeting, it would not come to fruition as the pressure would begin to mount on the former CDC visiting scientist.

David Thrower, a local father of an autistic son, traveled to the Sheraton Hotel to take a look at what ENSACP was doing, without realizing at the time that Poul Thorsen would soon become one of the most wanted fugitives in the United States or that he had been tossed out of Aarhus University.

In an email, Mr. Thrower said: "I recall the frustration of the trip and the poor attendance politically. About thirty of us went."[231]

What David Thrower didn't realize that at least three scientists in the group, including Dr. Simon Baron-Cohen from London, didn't attend the second ENSACP meeting, because Poul Thorsen's reputation as a fraud and alleged thief was growing more radioactive by the day.

Dr. Thorsen's second brainchild—the first being the defunct NANEA—in ENSACP, as he had envisioned it one night over wine and sex with Diana Schendel, wouldn't end up saving him, and he couldn't save it from being swallowed by the sinkhole of his negative reputation.

---

[230] Ibid.

[231] Email July 13, 2015: David Thrower, UK, to James O. Grundvig.

In the Spring 2010 newsletter of Irish Autism Action, Poul Thorsen who was in the photo of the group with the missing scientists from the second ENSACP meeting, on page 14, IAA announced:

> Initially the leadership of the project was jointly held by Dr. Poul Thorsen of Aarhus University, Denmark, and Dr. Alvaro Ramirez of Chiren Therapy Centre, Ireland. Following the resignation of Dr. Thorsen from Aarhus University and the subsequent withdrawal of that institution from the project, Irish Autism Action became the lead partner organization of the project, with Dr. Ramirez continuing as project leader.

Two and a half weeks after the ENSACP meeting in London, on March 9, 2010, Drexel University let go—read "fired"—Poul Thorsen as adjunct associate professor. Dismissed with little fanfare or explanation, Thorsen didn't even last one semester at the university in Philadelphia. Emory University finally cut ties with him that spring, followed by APA DSM-5 Work Group, as they couldn't keep the plutonium-hot Dr. Thorsen on its task force anymore, which would proceed to change the definition of autism spectrum disorders, perhaps in an attempt to somehow lower the autism incidence rate, and make the exploding world of childhood disabilities look rosier than it really was.

That is called the "flower of evil." Poul Thorsen centered the bloom of that budding flower, with the CDC executives being the petals.

## 2 4

# LIQUID METAL INDICTMENTS

The death spiral for Poul Thorsen was a one-two punch. Before the new managing director of Aarhus University struck him hard with a body blow in the January 2010 statement of "disownment," in March 2009 Østjllands (East Jutland) Police in Aarhus handed the Danish research scientist an *anklageskrift domsmandssag*—"indictment for criminal procedure."

The indictment spelled out the alleged tax crimes that Poul Thorsen committed from 2001 to 2005 at Odense and Aarhus, forcing him to hire a local attorney, Jan Schneider, a partner at the Tommy V. Christiansen law firm in Aarhus. In the Jutland police indictment, they tried to nail Thorsen with five counts of theft totaling 6.5 million DKK, or nearly $1 million USD.[232] Thorsen, it appeared, had major tax issues himself, like the former Nanean employees he screwed royally. The indictment was addressed to Thorsen's Briarlake

---

[232] Østjllands Police: Anklageskrift Domsmandssag—tax "indictment" Poul Thorsen, Atlanta, GA, March 16, 2009.

Road house in Atlanta, the one he paid for with CDC grant money back in 2006.

It appeared the alleged Danish thief didn't leave a forwarding address in Denmark. Good thing the East Jutland police were able to navigate the Internet to get Thorsen's new home address in America.

The two things worked in his advantage, other than hiring a top flight lawyer: first, OUH had two different accountants over the years since the alleged fraud began all the way back in 2001; and second, nearly a decade had passed by the time Thorsen's lawyer asked for discovery, won several postponements in court, and ultimately stretched the court case into late 2011-early 2012.

By the middle of summer 2010, the East Jutland police were overmatched. They were neither prepared for nor equipped to deal with attorney Jan Schneider and could not provide the smoking gun because the CDC, OUH, or Aarhus University partnership had never performed one single audit. Beyond the East Jutland police being embarrassed in the court of law and the court of public opinion, the second chief financial officer at Odense University Hospital in Niels Henning Poulsen fell on the sword, a sword meant for Poul Thorsen. Poul walked away from the alleged tax case free of punishment, yet was now trapped in his homeland with few job prospects.

From a detailed article written by journalist and engineer Jens Ramskov in the Copenhagen news magazine *Ingeniøren*, "The Engineer," he opened:

High Court rejects tax case for the next four million. kr. against Danish researcher, who is under suspicion in the United States for having rigged American research grants for recycling.

The former head of research at Aarhus University Poul Thorsen released apparently from a Danish tax case that could have given him a prison sentence and a tax fine of up to nearly four million.

"High Court has dismissed the indictment, because it is not accurate enough," wrote both (news bureau) Ritzau.dk & Ulla Danielsen on nbjour.wordpress.com.

The prosecution has in principle the opportunity to file a new indictment, but it is not known whether it will happen.

As previously discussed in the engineer has Attorney Sally Yates Quillian from Atlanta, USA, raised demands for the extradition of Poul Thorsen for fraud involving research funds for a million dollars, which he received from the US to research in Denmark, inter alia, Aarhus University.[233]

The other half of the one–two combination came from the United States. Poul Thorsen probably never anticipated the U.S. Department of Justice in the Southern District of Georgia would go hog-wild to catch him. But in DA Yates going for the jugular, the U.S. DOJ showed a lot more fang and bite than the East Jutland police. The order to investigate had to come from the CDC through the Department of Health and Human Services.

And it most likely had begun with then–CDC Director Julie Louise Gerberding, who knew when to pull the lever that got the CDC to contact Aarhus University—and not the other way around—about suspicious invoices. That had to occur right after Thorsen's last wire fraud and money laundering on Wednesday, October 29, 2008.

In a world that barely survived a total financial meltdown, someone had to be watching activity on Thorsen's five CDC Federal Credit Union bank accounts, either from inside the agency or from the IRS. Once all that money had been moved around in triple witching counts right before Halloween, all Dr. Gerberding had to do was make a call, wink, a nod to the right person, scribble a note on a Post-it, flash it,

---

[233] "Controversial Danish Researcher Released of Punitive Tax in Related Fraud," by Jens Ramskov, *Ingeniøren*, March 27, 2012.

and then rip it up, or simply tap someone's shoulder, drop a derogatory nickname for the Dane, and give a code word.

Having long planned for her exit before the next presidential election that November, Julie "Bioterror" Gerberding would let someone else go deal with the pursuit and fallout of the Poul Thorsen scandal. Sure, the Danish scientist was a wildcard. He abused the CDC's hospitality, sponsorship, and financial aid extended to him. But in the new darkness of the Great Recession, Gerberding, the master chess player, was three to four moves ahead of Poul Thorsen. She made sure Coleen Boyle and Marshalyn Yeargin-Allsopp would hold the fort down as she pulled the ripcord on her golden parachute, which would pay her millions in salary and stock in becoming the president of Merck's Vaccine Division in 2009. While she landed firmly on her feet with a massive pay raise, new powers, and ties with people at the FDA, CDC, and NIH, she knew how to manage and manipulate, too, and Dr. Thorsen began losing all kinds of support and potential jobs inside and outside of Denmark.

With a U.S. indictment, which would include twenty-two counts of wire fraud and money laundering—each count serving a ten-year sentence if convicted—Thorsen did the math and realized he would be in deep trouble if he stayed in the U.S. When he got word the FBI was leading the investigation in the U.S. in autumn 2010, Poul Thorsen had only one viable option, one get out of jail free card, and that was to bug out of Atlanta without selling his personal affects, such as the Harley, the cars, or the house.

Perhaps it was the ghost of Gerberding who tapped Poul on the shoulder and alerted him to leave the land of opportunity, the home of the American dream, and fly back to Denmark before he would be brought to court and asked to hand over his passport.

The ten-page indictment with twenty-two counts over a thirty-month period, draining money out of five CDC banks accounts that Thorsen opened had to include thousands of pages of affidavits, testimony, ledgers, emails, the forged invoices, and so much more in the intel sweep by the FBI. He would have little chance to survive such a court case.

Once the rising star and hero to the CDC problems over vaccine safety, MMR, and thimerosal, Poul Thorsen didn't so much go berserk like a Viking warrior as much as run off the rails. Untethered with no moral underpinnings and with no skills to build either a startup or research group, he took the fraud to the point of no return.

For Poul Thorsen, he blew by discretion. He couldn't contain his spending of the ill-gotten gains or tone down his behavior, or stop from sleeping with a coworker, or hold back from profusely exaggerating his talents. No, Poul Thorsen threw caution to the wind and then some. He burned more bridges than Napoleon's army in retreat at Waterloo. He used people, left them hanging. Forced his name into studies in which he did little to no work and slept with the help.

Perhaps the only thing I didn't uncover in the past year in researching the enigma of Dr. Thorsen was whether he had ever extorted or blackmailed anyone in his life. Since he was all about false airs and projecting strength, confidence, and erudition while possessing little of each quality himself, he was always about the money. Money, money, money. Whether he got paid in Danish crowns, U.S. dollars, Euros or bars of gold, Poul Thorsen was a money whore. His large down payments on the Harley Fat Boy and the four-bedroom house in the beautiful suburb of Atlanta confirmed that.

In Diana Schendel, he smelled more than the "musk of her hollows"—a line from a Kate Bush song. He smelled opportunity with the CDC. And with opportunity being his favorite word, he selfishly hogged it like a gluttonous swine rather than share it with his colleagues, the Naneans he nailed, and the students he failed to teach.

By 2012, the last known photograph of Poul—if it was him—is his back to a freelance photographer as he refused to answer the call of his name, or turn around and face the man speaking to him, or be man enough to show his own weathered, stressed face. And as that persistent photographer knocked on the door of the run-down row house in the suburb of Kolding, a city more spartan than Odense and directly to its west, Thorsen would not answer the door. He shriveled into the room he likely rented, as if he were Saddam Hussein after the American invasion in the Iraq War—find a remote farm, dig a deep hole, and go live in it in the fetal position. After all, he would certainly be familiar with the position after the two decades of studies on preterm deliveries and low-weight births. Poul Thorsen had come full circle and then some.

By the time his indictment was released to the public and press in mid April 2011 by the U.S. DOJ, two weeks before Poul's fiftieth birthday—time to celebrate, Poul; blow out the candles, Poul; eat the cake and smile, Poul; happy birthday, Poul!—the media in Denmark and the United States savaged him, and rightfully so.

He earned every derision, nasty comment, name-calling, and bile, hatred and bitterness by a broad spectrum of journalists, bloggers, and writers, many of them parents of autistic children. His scorched earth policy in living in the fast lane became the scorched earth that burned the soles of his feet.

With the tsunami of criticism spreading like wildfire in the forest of the Internet, the CDC, along with many other scientists who had long been bought off all came out and said as a chorus: "Yes, Poul is guilty of money fraud. But the science is solid. The science is good."

Contrary to the CDC staying "on message," making parents of brain damaged children appear as kooks with "anti-vaccine" labeling—the new Scarlet Letter—and saying with a Julie Gerberding smile that "the science is good, the vaccines are safe," the stark reality is quite different.

If Poul Thorsen's saga has proved anything, it's clear that the CDC suffers from "ROT": Redundant, Obsolete, and Trivial information.

The agency had suffered from ROT during the years it deliberately found "no link" between Agent Orange and sick Vietnam veterans, who only today are being recognized for the poisoning they suffered. Without rebuke from the White House or a full cleaning out by the next CDC director, in falling short of punishing CDC scientists, like Dr. Coleen Boyle who manipulated the Operation Ranch Hand data, the CDC grew a Teflon exterior, an impenetrable armor, while becoming part of the vaccine monolith. Boyle would be promoted all the way up to today being director at the CDC NCBDDD division, a place where Poul Thorsen got his grant funding start all the way back in 2000. Boyle and Thorsen deserve one another. He, a fugitive on the HHS's most wanted list; she, promoted and without a single reprimand.

It has become more than obvious that to stay or get ahead in the CDC, one would only have to drink its Kool-Aid, figure new ways to soften the blow of childhood disabilities, and tell the world and the parents that the Zombie Generation of spectrum children has always been a part of life, just under-diagnosed.

But then, the CDC and any pro-vaccine lover, with its bloated immunization schedule, have failed to show where even one tenth of the one million ASD kids are today in their parents' generation.

★   ★   ★

On Friday, May 29, 2015, I took the three-and-a-half-hour train ride from Copenhagen to Aarhus University wondering if I would meet Diana Schendel or speak with Poul Thorsen's lawyer Jan Schneider. Both were unknowns. So I made sure that I had a meeting that Friday noon that wouldn't raise any red flags that a nosey journalist from New York was poking around the university. I met with Fleming Svith, a tenured professor teaching investigative journalism at AU's School of Journalism—the first college dedicated to the science of information in Denmark—up the hill from the main campus and further up the road from NANEA's vacated office in a residential house.

Fleming and I made several phone calls over lunch, verifying that Poul Thorsen no longer worked at any of the major universities in Denmark and was out of the national hospital system—at least by means of the front door. Somehow he still has been able to snag coauthor credits on papers in 2014 and 2015, perhaps based in designs he purportedly did with other people's data many years before. In reality, he has been more or less out of work, out of the limelight, and stuck in his homeland by the U.S. extradition order that had never been executed—four years and counting. "The wrong paperwork has been filed by the United States," a Danish journalist told me over a beer.

In calling Diana Schendel twice—hearing her husky voice for the first time when I left a message to talk about Poul Thorsen—I took a taxi to NANA's old house at 17 Paludan Way. The red brick "funkis" villa had since been covered with three coats of beige paint, the platinum NANEA nameplate removed from the wall, and neither footprint nor fingerprint of Dr. Thorsen remained at the place where he abandoned his employees, leaving them on the hook with tax liabilities, as he flew first class to the U.S.

Next stop was AU's Department of Epidemiology building. Just before 3:00 pm, the taxi dropped me off and waited outside as I barged into the building. I talked to the receptionist on the ground floor; she pointed upstairs. I arrived at the second floor, but didn't find the German-American name on the faculty mailboxes. So I climbed the stairs of the barracks-type building up to the third floor, with the hallway door left ajar. Practically deserted on Friday afternoon, I found Diana Schendel's name on a label of her mailbox—empty. I asked one female scientist who walked by where Dr. Schendel's office was located, and she pointed around an alcove.

There, I stood before office No. 2.18 and read the nameplate: "Diana Schendel." Below her name, "Gill Rowland." I knocked on the door several times. No answer. Not a sound inside, nary a heartbeat nor the wisp of someone breathing. I slid my business card under the door with the very Danish sounding name of "James Ottar Grundvig" that had a New York City address. I had come a long way to rattle her cage.

I thought I would never hear from Poul Thorsen's lover again. But Diana would end up surprising me with her July 3rd cover-her-ass email that unwittingly introduced me to the executives of AU's School of Health. In believing her superiors might help her contain this journalist, she was mistaken. Instead, the eleven questions and backup docs I sent to the Dean of Health zeroed in on her "integrity of science."

On May 31, 2015, after I had the weekend to think about Poul Thorsen and Diana Schendel, I took a shorter train ride—thirty minutes west of Copenhagen—to a small, beautiful, historic coastal village on the fjord called Roskilde. As I walked from the station to the city square centered by a towering gothic cathedral, I could hear the roar of car engines zooming around down by the Roskilde Viking Museum on the water.

The straight walk down to the museum met a series of detours in fences, tents, and crowds cheering on the Denmark Historical Grand Prix race of souped-up Minis. I cut through a marina, passing replica Viking ships of all shapes and sizes, and strolled out a piece. I took out a sheet of paper I had printed and read the "Message from the Director" with a picture of the banal, short-haired, librarian-looking Coleen Boyle.

I glossed over her cheery mission statement and read the section, "The Future":

> The public health challenges that we face as a society today are complex, but our understanding of its intricacies has grown and continues to grow considerably. As the Director of the National Center on Birth Defects and Developmental Disabilities, I am proud of our work promoting the health of babies, children and adults and our continued progress in the pursuit ofimproved programs, research, and knowledge for the millions of Americans who live with birth defects, disabilities, and blood disorders. We are committed and will continue to evolve our programs to meet emerging public health needs, and to ensure community and partner engagement. Though our work is far from over, the foundation we have built strengthens our quest

for a better tomorrow. No one group can do this. It has to happen with CDC and with our partners. The Center's mission and CDC's mission is not complete until the most vulnerable in our nation are safer and healthier.[234]

I folded the paper and wondered who the true "master manipulator" really was. Was it the Danish opportunist Poul Thorsen? Or was Coleen Boyle the true master? And more significantly, should she take credit for developing the CDC study template that was designed to find "no association" between this or that while pointing to the bridge being out, when in fact it had been Photoshopped from the picture?

For a "puke lifer" like Boyle to waste Congress's money and time twice is mystifying. First finding no links that Agent Orange poisoned Vietnam veterans, and then erasing the links from liquid metal vaccines with autism—while getting promoted all the way up the food chain to director of a major healthcare agency division. The system is not only dull and broken but dying a slow, decaying death of irrelevancy.

Standing on the pier that beautiful Sunday afternoon, I gazed out the fjord, the stone longship-style museum on my right, and came to realize that like the three Viking ships that the Roskilde Norseman had buried 900 years ago in sending off their leaders on a voyage to Valhalla, the truth, the real story of what happened, doesn't stay buried forever. The kernel of truth, whether pushed up by a worm or by osmosis from underground, eventually makes its way to the surface, waiting to be exhumed or found, waiting for the first rays of light to dawn on its face in a long, long time.

When archaeologists excavated the Roskilde Viking ships in 1962,[235] Poul Thorsen was one year old. He grew up in nation that was growing in terms of education, technology, science, medicine,

---

[234] http://www.cdc.gov/ncbddd/aboutus/director.html
[235] https://en.wikipedia.org/wiki/Viking_Ship_Museum_(Roskilde)

GDP, sustainability, and above all social injustice. Infant Poul, who probably received two or three vaccines by the time he was five years old in 1966, had the future in front of him. One day Poul would throw it away in a trade for vanity, greed, and vainglory.

As I came to the end of the Thorsen road at the fjord of Roskilde, shutting out the drone of the Grand Prix racing behind me, I imagined seeing Viking longships sailing out to sea with their square sails dotting the blue water.

In that tranquil moment, I knew Poul Thorsen was no longer in charge of his history; info-archaeologists like myself were.

## 25

# MERCENARY SCIENTIST

In learning what under-the-radar Dr. Thorsen has been doing since he torched his own reputation and crashed his research career on the rocks in a flaming shipwreck while pouring kerosene on both in 2011-2012 with the U.S. Department of Justice's twenty-two-count indictment for money fraud, followed by the dismissed tax case from Odense University Hospital, I learned he not only was banging a Swedish woman on the side but living out in the open. But where has he lived for the past several years?

In his native Denmark, of course. No, not in the rural farmland he grew up in, leaving his late father's legacy of living a good, conservative, Christian farmer's legacy in the dust. No, not in Copenhagen, where his scientific incompetence, his lack of moral compass, and his penchant for self-promotion would have turned off too many of his peers. No, and not in Aarhus either, where Thorsen setup his shell research group NANEA, where all of his dirty dealings, theft of grant money designed for autism research, and his peddling of lies forced the managing director of Aarhus University in 2010 to sever all ties in a very rare, very unusual, very public statement that "disowned" the lousy, boring teacher in at least one former student's opinion.

No, Poul Bak Thorsen, who managed to get the CFO Niels Henning Poulsen of OUH fired months before his retirement over the tax evasion case he escaped, moved back to Odense to carry on his mercenary science, his gun for hire in a concealed manner at the very institution where he stole money from and manipulated the data. But I guess OUH—which did not return emails to comment on why it has rehired Dr. Poul Bak Thorsen—is clearly a failed institution with no ethical, moral, and scientific standards, not caring about the rule of law, while aiding and abetting a known fugitive.

Today, the incompetent doctor and science researcher, who manipulated vaccine safety data as a paid mercenary for the CDC, who left his former, underpaid, young employees of NANEA holding the tax liability bag with the Danish tax authorities, who has recycled more studies than this author has had hot meals, and who did "no work" on several of them while still receiving credit against the Vancouver Protocol for peer-reviewed studies and the standards held by the scientific journals themselves, moved to Odense where he earned his PhD in 1998 at the Southern District University at Odense.

Perhaps the real joke Thorsen has foisted on the million-plus autistic children in the United States, thumbed his nose at his former benefactor in the CDC, and flipped the middle finger at the U.S. Department of Justice's empty indictment and even lamer extradition filing (which has remained frozen since April 2011), has been him moving back to Odense. Today, the dirty Dane lives in a middle-income rowhouse on a nondescript street in the city. He rents from a local real estate property management company, which owns the house.

The biggest joke, however, has been played out for the past several years. After his April 2011 indictment went viral on the Internet, what could Poul Thorsen possibly do? He couldn't possibly work in the medical science research community after being shish kebobbed by Aarhus University's open letter of disowning him in 2010, could he? Not after leaving a debris field of bad, omitted, and manipulated data, could he? Not after having his name and reputation dragged through the Viking mud by the Danish news media in a relentless onslaught of articles and tales of theft and corruption from 2009 through 2012, could he? And what would the boy who grew up on a farm in the rural countryside do for a living, since the only thing Thorsen could ever milk was tax dollars and young people's commitment to science and learning and doing the right thing and CDC's grant money? Would Thorsen tend bar? Could he direct traffic in a sleepy town in the sticks? Would the man in his mid 50s, well past his prime, whore himself around in his favorite hobby of living off of and sleeping with lonely, desperate women? No. He did only the latter for a brief period.

Definitively, Odense University Hospital lacks character, has no ethical or moral standards, and is a glutton for punishment. Perhaps the research institution enjoys getting burned twice by the lousy, incompetent scientist. When I was in Denmark and called OUH inquiring about Dr. Poul Thorsen, the receptionist said his name didn't appear in her Rolodex. Thorsen's name also doesn't show up in a deep dive of all thirty-six research groups on OUH's website either.

Yet, through some nimble investigative research, I discovered Poul Thorsen does work at OUH in its Obstetrics and Gynecology Department. It does make sense, from his perspective: Continue the charade of being a skillful research scientist where he first sank his teeth a quarter century ago. The absolute need to confirm OUH's lunacy of allowing Poul Thorsen to work at its university research hospital came when the Female Email Avatar reached out to OUH directly in November 2015 when she emailed the main contact person.

A day later, OUH's contact person wrote this email reply:

"Dr. Poul Thorsen does not perform any research in Autism anymore, and he is not interested in contact."

Well, that was very noble of Thorsen to announced that after stealing millions of dollars in autism research money and manipulating data with the "Danish Studies" on behalf of his sponsor the CDC, which has allowed the autism epidemic in the United States to explode out of control, from 1 in 250 in 2000, when Thorsen secured his first research money from his friends in Atlanta, to 1 in 50 autism incidence rate in 2015 that he single-handedly has contributed to tens of thousands children being impaired with some form of the disorder on the spectrum the past fifteen years, including my son. He is a remarkable brute.

Thorsen might not be living large in Denmark, but he sure is making a living—still off CDC money, perhaps hush money?—and getting laid because he is not in prison and he is free to travel around borderless Scandinavia. Yet Thorsen is doing infinitely better than the parents of ASD children over the same stretch of time, including this author, who have been spending tens of thousands of dollars in treatment. Poul Thorsen's legacy is straightforward. Not only did he enrich himself, stain the institutions that aided and sponsored him, and deprive grant money meant for research, but he had a direct hand in the Vaccine Court's dismissal of more than 5,000 autism-by-thimerosal cases—which include my son—since those Masters (not the word I would use to call out the corrupt politicians) used the "Danish Studies" with Thorsen's name on them as the foundation for that dismissal.

Travesty doesn't begin to tell this sad tale of greed, maleficence, and corruption. The body is rotten, from head to toe, from Aarhus University and Odense University Hospital to the executives at the CDC, and particularly Dr. Coleen Boyle, director of the 2000 chartered National Center of Birth Defects and Developmental Disorder.

A review of the CDC-Denmark Program, "Collaboration Public Health Research," and its 2008–2012 financial records show the CDC has sent and continues to send tens of millions of U.S. tax dollars to continue to cook the data and backtest a national birth that is 95 percent white and doesn't at all mirror or reflect the diversity of the United States culturally diverse population. Why does the CDC send money abroad and offshore its research with a health database that in no way, size, shape or form resembles the 330 million Americans?

Perhaps the bigger questions are

Why hasn't the U.S. Department of Justice sent the papers to extradite Poul Thorsen to stand trial, convict him, and have the bastard research scientist spend the rest of his life in a U.S. federal prison?

Why does Aarhus University, after disowning Thorsen in 2010, go out of its way in 2015 to protect his lack of participation on the key "Danish Studies," which goes against that institution's own ethical and scientific standards and against the Vancouver Protocol?

Why does Odense University Hospital continue to hire the mercenary scientist, who burned that institution the first time around for hundreds of thousands of dollars? Like the CDC, those two leading Danish institutions have sold out, made a deal with the devil, and lowered their standards by any journeyman's view.

In September 2015, CDC announced it will fund an effort to combat "prescription overdose epidemic" to the tune of $20 million. From the newspaper UPI, the article opens:

> The U.S. Centers for Disease Control and Prevention announced today a $20 million program to work with 16 states in an effort to curtail the epidemic of opioid overdoses.
>
> Overdoses have quadrupled since 1999, according to the CDC.[236]

Since the CDC calls a quadrupling to 16,000 people dying of a prescription drug overdose today, then what about the quintupling—a factor of five times—the rate of autism incidence over the same span, from 1 in 250 to 1 in 50 today? We're not talking about 16,000 lives. We're talking about more than one million innocent babies who were born normal and fine and regressed.

---

[236] http://www.upi.com/Health_News/2015/09/04/CDC-to-fund-effort-against-prescription-drug-overdose-epidemic/6161441399926/

If the five times skyrocketing rate of autism in the United States doesn't alarm health officials and move both state and federal governments to action and call autism an epidemic, then at what rate will the government finally move to do something that is a burden on society in terms of costs for care, education, and health treatments, but also an opportunity cost since more than 90 percent of these children will not lead productive lives and join the work force.

One in ten babies born should wake up the next president of the United States to fire every executive at the CDC, open an investigation, and put the criminal scientists and manipulators to stand trial.

That sad day can't be too far off, as the epidemic has a lot of momentum and is clearly environmental with the neurotoxins.

How about one in five?

# EPILOGUE

# THE DATA DAM BREAKS

# 2 6

# THE FLOWER OF EVIL

The "Bravo Shot," heard around the world, was the first American test of a hydrogen bomb at Bikini Atoll. The 1954 blast, known as "Castle Bravo," was the "largest detonation the world had ever seen, one thousand times the power of the Hiroshima blast. "It was the morning, and I was fishing with my grandfather. He was throwing the net, and suddenly the silent bright flash—and then a force, the shock wave. Everything turned red—the ocean, the fish, the sky, and my grandfather's net. And we were 200 miles away from ground zero," recalled Tony De Brum. Today, the witness is an antinuclear activist and foreign minister of the Republic of the Marshall Islands.[237]

Years earlier, the last of the three American atomic bombs were detonated at Bikini Atoll on July 25, 1946, and it "blasted a water column 5,000 feet into the air."[238]

When the most powerful bombs in the world were detonated in tests, they were sights to behold, events to marvel at. They were

---

[237] "Marshall Islands Moment," Editorial of the *New York Sun*, April 28, 2015.
[238] "How the Summer of Atomic Bomb Testing Turned the Bikini Into a Phenomenon," Jennifer Le Zotte Smithsonian.com, May 21, 2015.

bright flashes of yellow-orange, their cloud cores ascending, towering, the mushroom clouds spreading out, blasting through air molecules, burning oxygen, while stilling the land and sea and sky around them in immense silence. So powerful was the bright light of a nuclear bomb blast that a blind girl once saw the flash of the Trinity detonation from many miles away.[239]

Beautiful. Awe-inspiring. Memorable at first, a nuclear bomb belies its true nature as a beast. Windstorms and superheated fires following in the wake were just the beginning of the hell that would soon arrive for anyone living near—or as far away as 200 miles—with the nuclear, plutonium, and radioactive dust that would rain down, drifting on the air currents. The "flower of evil" masked the true nature of being vaporized, turned into ash, or poisoned with cancer from the inside out by the fallout.

Without having conducted any real safety testing or clinical trials— as opposed to backtesting data and running various methods to ensure goals are met—when U.S. Congressman Bill Posey asked CDC Dr. Coleen Boyle at the 2012 Congressional hearing whether any studies had ever been done to compare "vaccinated versus unvaccinated" infants, she replied, "No."

The CDC, with its national "Listening Sessions," SEED, and other programs intended to show how the agency cares about children, their problems, and the concerns of parents, is projecting a false hope and optimism that the Centers for Disease Control is a bright, shining beacon of health and well-being that has been tasked to help several million American children with tics, autism, and other learning disabilities. CDC's flower of evil is not a plant that grows outside its Druid Hills headquarters in Atlanta, but the great lengths it has gone to and the costs it has burned through to keep the veil that vaccines are safe intact and that the metals that are unnatural to the human

---

[239] http://www.pbs.org/wgbh/americanexperience/features/primary-resources/truman-bombtest/

body, like mercury and aluminum compounds, don't pose a threat to babies, infants, children, and pregnant women jabbed over and again in a ceaseless, out of control, bloated vaccine program.

In fall of 2015, a peer-reviewed study—"Toxicopathological Effects of the Sunscreen UV Filter, Oxybenzone (Benzophenone-3), on Coral Planulae and Cultured Primary Cells and Its Environmental Contamination in Hawaii and the U.S. Virgin Islands," by C. A. Downs et al.—showed what the accumulative effect of a micro chemical could do in destroying a vastly larger ecosystem than the humans that apply sunscreen to protect their skin from sunburn, the weathered look, and the potential effects of some people getting skin cancer. That point was driven home in a newspaper article:

It only takes one part of oxybenzone per 62 trillion parts of water to have a deleterious effect on the reef. In the studied areas, concentrations were 12 times as high.

Oxybenzone works to disrupt coral DNA, causing the coral to encase itself in its own skeleton and die.

Oxybenzone is found in 3,500 sunscreen brands, and if you're worried that a compound that can change coral DNA might change yours too, concerns have been raised about that.[240]

If the cumulative effect of single chemical compound in sunscreen, with only "one part per 62 trillion parts of water . . . have a deleterious effect" on a coral reef, such as making the marine plant vulnerable to bleaching, what does the accumulative effect of micro amounts of mercury and aluminum have on the development of a much smaller-than-a-reef baby's nervous system, lungs, and brain in a human's most vulnerable phase, in the womb or right after birth?

[240] "Study shows sunscreen is killing coral reefs in tourist areas," Katie Dowd, www.sfgate.com, October 21, 2015.

It doesn't take a rocket scientist to understand the impact that small amounts of human-made, human-produced, and human-released compounds have on the earth's atmosphere, ozone layer, oceans, land, marine, plant, and wildlife can also affect the vulnerable human baby and infant.

There is no leap of faith in that. Then why has mainstream media, without their own independent, investigative research into the leading cause of autism in too many, too soon, and too toxic vaccines, bought the CDC tripe that vaccines are safe, no matter how many, served at any age? Not only does it make little sense, defying the logic of a critical thinking of an educated adult, it deflates any argument that mankind, through pollution and climate change, are damaging the planet.

The U.S. has bought into the success of the Teflon CDC, who has killed the messenger, hyped false panics around H1N1 and other so-called pandemics including the great measles outbreak in Disneyland, and continued to dress up and press people to take the flu shot when it protects against the wrong strain of flu. From Reuters:

> A sampling of flu cases so far this season suggests the current flu vaccine may not be a good match for the seasonal flu strain currently circulating in the United States, the U.S. Centers for Disease Control and Prevention on Wednesday.[241]

The flowers of evil that populate the CDC's garden are mercury in the form of ethylmercury and at least three different types of aluminum salts as adjuvants that are used as "an ingredient of a vaccine that helps create a stronger immune response in the patient's body."[242] The CDC is also the holder of the HPV vaccine patent, which the

---

[241] "CDC says Flu Shots may not be Good Match for 2014–15 Virus," Julie Steenhuysen, Reuters, Dec. 3, 2014.

[242] http://www.cdc.gov/vaccinesafety/Concerns/adjuvants.html

FDA recently approved and which could double the amount of aluminum adjuvant.[243]

The CDC's flower of evil is making harmful ingredients that get injected into babies without true clinical trials on safety ever being done. The so-called bedrock "Danish Studies" the CDC has hung its flimsy hat on as "solid science," in which they paid the study troll Poul Thorsen through the nose to accomplish, has been demolished in this book as cooked and manipulated.

Instead of worrying about the healthcare of children and how vaccines have damaged a growing subpopulation of children with an array of disorders, former CDC Director Julie Gerberding, now president of Merck's Vaccine Division, sold 38,368 shares of Merck stock as an "office," at $60.99/share, or $2,340,064 on May 8, 2015.[244] It was the second largest sale in dollars of Merck shares in the month of May.

As the "Golden Girl of Bioterrorism" tapped into her golden parachute, she, like many other executives at the CDC, FDA, NIH, IOM, NIH, and NCBDDD, has enjoyed the riches of the vaccine industry's great windfall while transferring the costs of her deceit onto American taxpayers in general and children on the spectrum in particular, while also harming the future potential of the U.S. workforce by creating a brain drain of zombie children, who will never participate in the job market, and thus become a burden to their families and society instead of a taxpayer.

As Dr. Julie Gerberding took care of herself, and made sure she rewarded Coleen Boyle for twice not finding any association in the Agent Orange debacle and the autism epidemic, she left Diana Schendel to her own devices. When the full story about Poul Thorsen's alleged wire fraud and money laundering activities surfaced, the CDC

---

[243] "Aluminum: Has The FDA Got It All Wrong?" Catherine J. Frompovich, www.Vactruth.com, January 2, 2012

[244] https://finance.yahoo.com/q/it?s=MRK+Insider+Transactions

had little choice but to give Schendel the two-year probationary letter of reprimand that would make firing her easy by threatening to kill her federal pension.

Diana Schendel's only viable option was to take up Poul Thorsen's suggestion that she move to Denmark in 2013 and continue her work in autism in the epidemiology department at Aarhus University. With the transfer in place, Schendel became a full-time professor at the university the following year.

In trying to interview her, to learn more about who she was and what motivated her to move to Denmark to live out the rest of her life, I created a Female Email Avatar to coax her into doing an interview, an interview that I would never write or publish. But because my trip to Denmark had been planned in advance and she would end up attending the INSAR autism conference in Utah the week before I arrived after Memorial Day, I never got the chance to email her the dozen questions I had planned.

As the Female Email Avatar, I set up a bait email address, adding the feminine touches of having a woman's signature and pale blue background. I couldn't telegraph that I was a man or of Scandinavian heritage or from media-driven New York City. And I definitely couldn't share with her that I was a father of an autistic boy.

After a few email exchanges to open the communication channel between the Female Email Avatar and Diana Schendel, her auto-email replied on May 13, 2015:

"I am out of the office and with limited email access. I will reply to your message when I return 19 May 2015. Thank you for your patience. Diana."

In sending her an email the middle of the following week, Diana Schendel finally responded on May 26, 2015, or when I was already in Denmark, writing:

"I am not sure I can help you. Based on the description of your article that you sent earlier, I was doubtful that I could contribute. We can chat if you want, but I thought I would send you a warning first. Best, Diana."

Diana and the Female Email Avatar were becoming fast friends. With a little more push to "chat" and answer a "dozen questions," she replied on May 28, 2015, or the Thursday before I would take the train from Copenhagen to Aarhus the next day to try to meet and interview her. She wrote:

> I have a background in anthropology but have not worked in the anthropology field as a professional. My studies on children with impairments are looking at causes of their disabilities (like the causes of cerebral palsy or autism) using medical data, and not with any examination of children's behavior or lifestyle or family environment. So, I am not sure I have the relevant expertise to help you, but you can send me some questions as an exploratory step if you like. Best, Diana.

With the emphasis being mine with her line "not with any examination of children's behavior (which was understood) or lifestyle or family environment." It was the last word, "environment," as if she didn't do family health studies and histories, as if she didn't realize the pollution from the environments she researched and analyzed had an impact on the children who became ill or worse. So I wondered what the word "environment" meant to an anthropologist. What did it mean to the PhD who took her first real post-graduate job with the Woburn, Massachusetts, WEBS project? That epidemiological study on the two toxic wells, which had become a Superfund Site, was all about the environment and the "family environment," too, with her interviewing the families about the children who came down with rare cancers in the cancer clusters that haunted the small town north of Boston.

When she went to the CDC to work under the direction of Coleen Boyle, who was the master of finding no linkages between industrial dioxin spraying of Agent Orange and the environment of the Vietnam War, Schendel was on the road to being indoctrinated in the CDC.

And that spurred her to study autism and vaccines separately, as if they existed on separate planets. But there was nothing more environmental than the mercury and aluminum in vaccines and the harm those metal compounds have done to the children the past quarter of a century.

Dr. Diana Schendel was either blind to it or submitted to toeing the line her two decades at the CDC. She slept with Poul Thorsen, so it had to be the latter.

# 27

# WEAPONIZATION OF GOVERNMENT

With the United States split down the middle of political classes in Washington, the gridlock provided cover for politicians and agency heads alike. One just had to pick up a newspaper, read an online blog, or watch the news and they would have seen the IRS target groups it didn't like in order to harass them, fine them, and shut them down; or seen that the ObamaCare website and rollout was in a bottom-feeding class in terms of total incompetence; or seen that the mammoth hack of government employees at the Office of People Management (time to rename that agency, just like President Obama did in the failed response during the 2010 BP oil spill) that exposed private records of 24 million federal workers' personal information, including home addresses, social security numbers, what agencies they worked for, and so on to Chinese military hackers.

Like the cancer and excesses affecting much of the federal government, CDC has long operated in an age of inaction, misdirection, cover-ups, and protectionism.

That model twentieth century is wholly different than the American people who live and work in society in the Age of Mobility, Big Data,

Transparency, and Open Source and Shared Economy. Government failure has never looked so good.

The weaponization of government goes far beyond the militarization of state and local police departments during the 2014 Ferguson and 2015 Baltimore riots. It's about taking over your lives at a very young age. And vaccines are the first place to start. Centers for Disease Control has done a masterful job, together with the Dept. of Health and Human Services, in not extraditing fugitive Poul Thorsen. But it fumbled in other keys areas. Namely, the mass panic and piss-poor communication in the Ebola outbreak, which showed the CDC was woefully unprepared to explain to the American people in plain language what was transpiring in Western Africa or how the disease left the continent. CDC Director Tom Frieden couldn't articulate what Ebola was either. Why not? He couldn't say where it came from. How come? Or how the virulent disease was transmitted. Why, for God's sake? Or how Ebola ended up in West Africa, after showing up forty years ago in northern Congo.

Pathetic is the only word to describe CDC's Tom Frieden. In the private sector, he would have been fired after fumbling the message on Ebola with the American people.

By mid October 2014, the low point of the CDC's mishandling of the Ebola crisis took a turn for the worse in a negative public relations disaster that went viral, spreading faster than the not fully understood, poorly articulated disease, when the New York Post published the fabulous headline: "Air Ebola: Frantic Hunt for 132 Passengers."[245]

The headline below a picture of an airplane taking off was the final nail in the coffin for CDC's Tom Frieden to be the face of calm reassurance on TV and at press conferences. As good a microbiologist Dr. Frieden might have been, he was no Julie "Dr. Anthrax" Gerberding, who knew exactly what to say to the public, and when and how to

---

[245] "Air Ebola: Frantic Search for 132 Passengers," New York Post cover story, Oct. 16, 2014.

take charge during a crisis or disease outbreak. But she had moved on to become president of Merck's Vaccine Division. President Obama had little choice—but he did have one, which really had never been done before, at least not going back to the CDC's epidemiology studies of Agent Orange in the 1980s: Fire the director.

Instead, President Obama went out of his way to calm fears of Americans as the sick passenger passed the Ebola virus onto a couple nurses tending to the patient in a quarantine ward at a Dallas hospital. But the semi-containment suits and other outdated CDC protocols to protect the nurses were as flawed as Tom Frieden's failed ability to communicate the agency's message and mistakes to the general public.

To douse the contagion of fear from spreading more than it already moved with the media, President Obama made the soft decision, the lighter choice and invented a new post in the "Ebola Czar." The czar would work out of Washington, DC, far from the Atlanta headquarters, where Dr. Tom Frieden and the CDC were losing on two fronts. They got routed in the court of public opinion and had deep trouble containing, let alone extinguishing, the Ebola crisis in 2014.

And who became the president's choice for mouthpiece to replace Tom Frieden? Ron Klain. And if Mr. Klain failed to communicate the Ebola crisis, then the American people might have started calling him "Ron Blame."

"President Barack Obama has appointed longtime insider Ron Klain to coordinate the administration's global response to the Ebola epidemic, a White House official confirmed. The move came just hours after a Texas nurse diagnosed with Ebola after treating a patient with the disease was moved from Dallas to the National Institutes of Health Clinical Center in Bethesda, Maryland."[246]

Pissed, like the rest of the U.S. citizens at the time, feeling we didn't have clear answers on all that was being done by the CDC to stem the

---

[246] "Obama Appoints Ron Klain as Ebola Czar," Zeke J. Miller, *Time Magazine*, Oct. 17, 2014.

avalanche of fear or stop the spread of the lethal disease, this author no longer trusted either the White House (same as fumbling the BP oil spill) or the CDC to provide clarity. Instead of waiting for the mainstream press to come out with news, as it did in January 2015, that the Ebola outbreak began with migratory bats transferring the virus to a baby in Sierra Leone, I spent two days researching the short but fascinating history of Ebola. There are four strains of the virus—the one from the Philippines isn't harmful to humans yet—which first showed in Central Africa in 1976, the same summer that AIDS arrived supposedly with gay sailors on "Operation Sail" to celebrate the United States' bicentennial. I learned everything I needed to know about the disease without the overhyped fear that Ebola would break out on the streets of New York City. Was that a coincidence?

In an article I published a few days after Ron Klain was named Ebola Czar, I wrote in the *Epoch Times* Opinion section:

"Four decades after the first outbreak of the Ebola virus in Central Africa, misconceptions and misinformation about the disease abound. No one from the CDC to the WHO has been able to articulate the scope of the problem well."[247]

In a take-no-prisoners article, I, by myself as a freelance journalist with no staff, had outmaneuvered the clearly overpaid scientists and PR professionals at the CDC, as well as the White House, in articulating what Ebola was, how it spread, whether it could turn into a pandemic (no, it could not), and so on. And yet, for his increase in six-figure salary, bonuses, perks, benefits, and pension that Dr. Tom Frieden was rewarded to become director of the CDC, or the quiet the Ebola virus had instilled on the newly appointed Ebola Czar in Ron Klain, I figured out what they couldn't tell or express to the American people for another ninety days. Pathetic. And they supposedly represented

---

[247] "The Ebola bats: How Deforestation Unleashed the Deadly Outbreak," James O. Grundvig, the *Epoch Times*, Oct. 20, 2014.

the frontline of defense in case of a true global pandemic running through societies around the world.

To hammer home the CDC's flaws in mishandling the outbreak, a blog on science nailed the precarious situation American citizens were:

> The Ebola situation is testing the world's best infectious disease team, the Centers for Disease Control and Prevention (CDC), at its ability to perform crisis management. While the immediate threat in the United States appears to be receding, it is far from clear that we're up to facing a stronger test.[248]

CDC Whistleblower Dr. Bill Thompson brought the question of autism to Tom Frieden standing on the proscenium under the klieg lights.

Thompson said:

> He does have clean hands. But I don't know where he stands on all of this. I really don't. I do think this. I do think Frieden, I think he has closed himself off from all of this and avoids this and says this is Coleen Boyle and uh Melinda Wharton's problem.[249]

The CDC had other problems beyond Friedman's failure to communicate, and it started with the mishandling of anthrax spores.

All of that under Dr. Frieden's watch. Dr. Julie Louise Gerberding must have smiled. Her golden parachute sure did.

---

[248] http://www.realclearscience.com/2014/10/24/how_the_cdc_fumbled_its_ebola_response_261616.html

[249] *Vaccine Whistleblower: Exposing Autism Research Fraud at the CDC,* by Kevin Barry, Esq., Skyhorse Publishing 2015, pg. 21.

# 28

# THE VACCINE DEEP STATE

The monolith of the CDC-FDA-NIH is supposed to be separated by a divide with the big pharma vaccine producers. But since the NIH rejected the Swedish scientist's brief that all thimerosal should be removed from vaccines in 1992, there has been little to no separation of powers, policies, messaging, or enforcement between government oversight and industry manufacturers.

The separation of church and state doesn't exist anymore in the vaccine industry, not with Vaccine Court squashing all comers, the Dick Armey "Lilly Rider" slipped into the 2002 Homeland Security Act, and the FDA's approval to double the doses of aluminum adjuvants in several vaccines.

Vaccines today are part of a program rife with ROT and deception.

In a September 2007 hearing by the Committee on Health, Education, Labor and Pensions for "Thimerosal and Autism Spectrum Disorders: Alleged Misconduct by Government Agencies and Private Entities," the executive summary naturally found no misconduct on behalf of the CDC—this was a case of one hand washing the other. It read:

While the five studies in question may have varying connections to the CDC and/or vaccine manufacturers, their value to consideration of an alleged link between vaccines and autism is a matter for the experts of the ISR Committee, and not for Congress.[250]

What the findings got wrong by one half of the government to keep Congress in its place, since they were not qualified to review scientific data, as good as the "experts" that false assertion was nothing more than a ruse, a smokescreen. What Congress needs to do is evaluate the human side of this tragedy and ongoing fraud. It has nothing to do with science—no scientific expertise is required, just the nose to follow the money.

It has everything to do with corruption, cover-up, relentless greed, pulling the ripcords on golden parachutes, shielding vaccine makers from harm, all while exposing millions of babies, children, and people around the world to great harm.

Congress needs only to examine agendas, follow the email trails, and begin to pull the weeds that have infested the CDC, FDA, and NIH lawn, removing all of the ROT as they should have done in 1990 with the Agent Orange finding. Had they done that, then maybe Coleen Boyle would have become a librarian instead of the director of NCBDDD, and Diana Schendel would have done good collaborative studies instead of the studies that had a fixed objective to show no association, and maybe Poul Thorsen wouldn't have been invited to come to the CDC as a visiting professor or been able to secure funding for the cooperative agreements because the "hunt for good data" never would have taken place.

But that is a story meant for a parallel universe, where moral decency and real scientific integrity, real scientific honesty—absent

---

[250] *Thimerosal and Autism Spectrum Disorders: Alleged Misconduct by Government Agencies and Private Entities,* September 2007 Executive Summary, pg. 5.

at CDC and its partner Aarhus University—would rule the day, and a "less is more" approach to vaccines would make for a safer immunization program.

Why is it so hard for mainstream media, independent journalists, and government officials on both sides of the aisle to grasp the dangers of micro small toxins? If they believe that the unseen greenhouse gas particulates and molecules can superheat the world and change climate, why is it so hard to believe that traces of mercury and aluminum in vaccines have harmed so many once promising, healthy children for the past two decades?

If a grown man can die from a tiny amount of venom in a bee sting, then why is it so hard to believe that trace amounts of metals in babies who weight from seven to twenty-five pounds can have adverse reactions to being injected with toxins, especially when all of their bodies—from the central nervous and immune systems to the brain and lungs—are under development?

"Less is more" is a motto that our politicians need to take up with the Vaccine Deep State and rein it in. If they cannot do it, don't have the will to do it, don't have the balls to do it, or won't expend the political capital to do it, a tipping point will soon one day force there hand.

When will that occur? When 1 in 40 babies are born on the spectrum? One in 25 babies born? How about 1 in 10? Will the rate of autism incidence in the United States have to soar to that sky high number for our government to react and belatedly realize that the autism epidemic has been real all along, and its long-over due to do something about it?

The next generation of Americans, who will be born over the next decade, is awaiting your call to action. Will you act?

# BIBLIOGRAPHY

101st Congress Report: *The Agent Orange Coverup: A Case of Flawed Science and Political Manipulation, the Twelfth Report by the Committee on Government Operations*, together with Dissenting Views, August 9, 1990, (Washington, DC), pp. 1–33, 43.

*Air Ebola: Frantic Search for 132 Passengers,* New York Post cover story, (New York, NY) October 16, 2014.

Ankara Media Reaction Report, Cabal Press Briefing, "Vaccine Crisis in the U.S.," provided by Wikileaks.org (Stockholm, Sweden) August 18, 2005.

Assessment of the Recommendations of the Advisory Committee on Immunization Practices (ACIP)," Journal of American Physicians and Surgeons, (Tucson, Arizona) Vol. 11, No. 2, Summer 2006.

Autism Dublin 2010 – *European Autism Action 2020: A Strategic Health Care Plan,* slide 10.

Autism Speaks, "Pilot Study Grants to Poul Thorsen," 2002 Research Awards.

David M. Ayoub, MD, and F. Ed Yazbak, MD, "*Influenza Vaccination During Pregnancy*" A Critical Assessment of the Recommendations of *the Advisory Committee on Immunization Practices (ACIP)*, Journal of American Physicians and Surgeons, Vol. 11, No. 2, Summer 2006.

Barry, Kevin, Editor, "Vaccine Whistleblower: Exposing the Autism Research Fraud at the CDC," Skyhorse Publishing (New York, NY) 2015: Transcript 1, May 8, 2014, p. 9, Transcript 2, May 24, 2014, pp. 21, 26.

Berezow, Alex, "How the CDC Fumbled Its Ebola Response," USA Today (United States), October 24, 2014.

Blaxill, Mark and Dan Olmsted, "A New Paradigm for a Post-Imperial World: Poul Thorsen's Mutating Resume," Age of Autism, (Boston, Massachusetts) April 5, 2010.

Blaxill, Mark, "SafeMinds' Mark Blaxill Testimony at Autism Hearing: Testimony of Mark Blaxill Board Member, SafeMinds Before the Committee on Oversight and Government Reform US House of Representatives," Age of Autism, (Boston, Massachusetts) November 29, 2012.

Blaxill, Mark, Director SafeMinds, "Danish Thimerosal-Autism Study in Pediatrics: Misleading and Uninformative on Autism-Mercury Link," Safeminds.org, (Boston, Massachusetts) September 2, 2003.

Blaxill, Mark, Editor at Large Age of Autism, email to James O. Grundvig, "Press Inquiry," (Boston, Massachusetts) July 19, 2015.

Blaxill, Mark, Letters to the Editor: "Concerns Continue Over Mercury and Autism," American Journal of Preventative Medicine, (Boston, Massachusetts) 2004, 26(1).

Blomgren, Berit Agneta, House Sale Advertisement, Center in Danderyd (Stocksund, Sweden) September 1, 2009, p. 35.

J. Bonhoeffer, et al., *The Brighton Collaboration: addressing the need for standardized case definitions of adverse events following immunization (AEFI)*, Elsevier, Vaccine 21, 2002, pg. 298.

Boyle, Coleen, Biography: Coleen Boyle, Director National Centers for Birth Defects and Developmental Disabilities, Centers for Disease Control, (Atlanta, Georgia).

Boyle, Coleen, email to Frank DeStefano: "Comments on Analysis," Centers for Disease Control, (Atlanta, Georgia) April 25, 2000.

Boyle, Coleen, email to Jose Cordero, "Autism Thimerosal Paper – Cover Letter," National Centers for Birth Defects and Developmental Disabilities, Centers for Disease Control (Atlanta, Georgia), November 26, 2002.

Briarlake Road NE, Atlanta Georgia, 30345, Trulia.com, "Home Details," (Atlanta, Georgia) 2015.

Briarlake Road NE, Atlanta Georgia, 30345, Zwillow.com, "Home Details," (Atlanta, Georgia) 2015.

Brøndby Community, "Brøndby Kommune markerede 70 års dagen for Danmarks Befrielse," [70ᵗʰ Anniversary of Denmark's Liberation from WWII], (Brøndby , Denmark) March 5, 2015, http://www.brondby.dk/Service/Nyheder/2015/05/Broendby-Kommune-markerede-70-aars-dagen-for-Danmarks-Befrielse.

*Case definitions of adverse events following immunization (AEFI)*, Elsevier, Vaccine 21

CDC Federal Credit Union, "Membership Eligibility," Centers for Disease Control (Atlanta, Georgia). https://www.cdcfcu.com/Online-Services/Join.

Center for Birth Defects and Developmental Disorders, Centers for Disease Control, (Atlanta, Georgia).

Centers for Disease Control online, "Vaccine Safety," (Atlanta, Georgia).

Centers for Disease Control, "Autism Spectrum Disorders: Data Statistics," National Centers for Disease Control, "Scientific Review of Vaccine Safety Datalink Information," Simpsonwood Retreat Center (Norcross, Georgia), June 7-8, 2000, pp. 151, 166, 247.

Centers for Disease Control, "Technical Review Evaluation Report" to Danish Medical Research Council, (Atlanta, Georgia) November 17, 2003.

*Congressional Research Service, Report RL31649, Homeland Security Act of 2002: Tort Liability Provision, Henry Cohen, American Law Division,* provided by Wikileaks.org (Stockholm, Sweden) May 9, 2000, p. CRS-10.

Conradsen, Marie Louise, "The Cancer Center that Never Was: The Organization of Danish Cancer Research 1949-1992," Doctoral Thesis, Copenhagen Business School (Copenhagen, Denmark), 1992, pp. 202, 205, 233, 234.

Cowlishaw, Kitt and Terri Dowty, Editors, "Home Educating Our Autistic Spectrum Children: Paths are Made by Walking," Jessica Kingsley Publishers, (Philadelphia, Pennsylvania), September 15, 2001, p. 289.

Dales, Loring, email to Diane Simpson, CDC, "DTP Coverage and Autism Caseload on Calif. – Time Trend Data," California Dept. of Health Services, (Berkley, California) June 8, 2001.

Danielsen, Ulla, "Danish Odense University Hospital Lost Four-Five Million DKK by Poul Thorsen's Research Grants," NBJour, (Copenhagen, Denmark) January 7, 2012

Danielsen, Ulla, "Dec 23 1999: Cerebal [sic] Palsy Letter from U.S. CDC to Ib Terp, DK," NBJour online blog, (Copenhagen, Denmark) December 23, 2014.

Danielsen, Ulla, "Researcher, Not University Hospital, Accounted to U.S. CDC," NBJour, (Copenhagen, Denmark) February 15, 2012.

Denmark Culture online: http://www.everyculture.com/Cr-Ga/ Denmark.html

Department of Homeland Security, Homeland Security Act of 2002 (H.R. 5005), November 25, 2002, pp. 472-73.

Deutsche Welle, "Jewish Victim of Copenhagen Shooting Buried," February 18, 2018.

Dowd, Katie. "Study shows sunscreen is killing coral reefs in tourist areas," SFgate.com, (San Francisco, California) October 21, 2015.

Duke University Medical Center, "Evolution Of The Human Appendix: A Biological 'Remnant' No More," Science Daily, August 21, 2009.

Eberlin Reporting Services, Silver Springs, MD transcribed "Workshop on Aluminum in Vaccines," May 11, 2000, pp. 1, 23, 36, 59, 63, 64, 65, 187, 191.

Eberlin Reporting Services, Silver Springs, MD transcribed "Workshop on Aluminum in Vaccines," May 12, 2000, pp. 126, 146.

Editorial: "A Time of Change at the CDC, Infectious Diseases," The Lancet, Vol. 2, August 2002.

Edmundson, Lauren, "Polio To Be Eradicated By 2018?" The Disease Daily, April effective Date 12-22-1999.

Eli Lilly and Company, Material Safety Data Sheet: "Thimerosal," (Indianapolis, Indiana),

Elkins, Kathleen, "The practice legendary tycoon Andrew Carnegie credits for his riches can be used by anyone," Business Insider, (New York, NY) June 26, 2015.

Emory University Newsletter, "Departments, Epidemiology," (Atlanta, Georgia) Spring 2008.

Enzi, Senator Michael B., U.S. Senate, Committee on Health, Education, Labor and Pensions, "Thimerosal and Autism Spectrum Disorders: Alleged Misconduct by Government Agencies and Private Entities," (Washington, DC) September 2007, Executive Summary p. 5.

EPI News, June 11, 2010.

European Network of Surveillance on Autism and Cerebral Palsy (ENSACP), Minutes of the

Meeting, Transcript, (Wolfheze, Netherlands), June 6-7, 2009, p.4.

European Network of Surveillance on Autism and Cerebral Palsy (ENSACP), Minutes of the Meeting, Transcript, (London, UK), February 20-21, 2010.

Exchange Rates "U.S. Dollars to Danish Krone 2012" (New York, New York) 2012.

F-D-C Reports, Inc., "The Pink Sheet," 46 (23): T&G-3, June 4, 1984.

F-D-C Reports, Inc., "The Pink Sheet," 48 (30): 3-4, July 28, 1986.

FDA, CFR – Code of Federal Regulations, Title 21 http://www.
accessdata.fda.gov/scripts/cdrh/cfdocs/cfcfr/CFRSearch.
cfm?fr=610.15.

Feller, Stephen, "CDC to fund effort against prescription drug overdose epidemic Opioid overdoses in the United States have quadrupled since 1999," United Press International, (Washington, DC),
September 4, 2015.

Flyvbjerg, Allan, Dean of Health at Aarhus University, email to James O.
Grundvig, "Poul Thorsen," (Aarhus, Denmark) July 13, 2015.

Flyvbjerg, Allan, Dean of Health, Aarhus University, Letter to James
O. Grundvig: "Concerning Your Letter Regarding Poul Thorsen,"
(Aarhus, Denmark) August 20, 2015.

Frompovich, Catherine J., "Aluminum: Has The FDA Got It All
Wrong?" Vactruth.com, (United States) January 2, 2012.

Funch, Sanne Maja, "When the Agitator Came to the University,"
Information.DK, (Copenhagen, Denmark) March 13, 2010.

Furlow, Bryant, "The Acinetobacter Threat," Overseas Civilian
Contractors online.

General Accounting Office, "Agent Orange Studies: Poor Contracting
Practices at Centers for Disease Control Increased Costs,"
(Washington, DC), September 28, 1990, pp. 1, 2, 15.

Gerberding, Ancestory.com: http://www.ancestry.com/name-origin?
surname=gerberding

Gerberding, Julie, President Vaccine Division, Merck & Company,
"Trading Shares," Yahoo.com (Mountainview, California) May 8,
2015.

Gianakaris, Niki, media relations Drexel University, email to James O.
Grundvig, "Poul Thorsen," (Philadelphia, Pennsylvania) April 15,
2015.

Glass, Roger I., "The 8th Richard J. Duma/NFID Annual Press
Conference and Symposium on Infectious Diseases, "Norovirus:
An Emerging Viral Pathogen," PR Newswire (New York, NY),
July 16, 2003.

Grandjean, Philippe, Biography: Philippe Grandjean, Harvard University, (Cambridge, Massachusetts) http://www.hsph.harvard.edu/philippe-grandjean/.

Granstrom, Marta, email to Diane Simpson, Centers for Disease Control, Atlanta, Georgia, "Vaccine Preservatives," Medical Products Agency, (Uppsala, Sweden), June 22, 2001.

Greenwald, Glenn, "Vital Unresolved Anthrax Questions and ABC News," Salon.com, (London, UK) August 1, 2008.

Grundvig, James O., "The Ebola bats: How Deforestation Unleashed the Deadly Outbreak," *Epoch Times*, (New York, NY) October 20, 2014.

Grundvig, James, "We Lost the Propaganda War: From Twitter to Denmark," *Epoch Times*, (New York, NY) March 12, 2015, Section A-11.

*Guide to Department of Anthropology*, Penn State University, (State College, Pennsylvania) 1989-90.

Harley Davidson Motorcycle, "Screaming Boy," specifications, Classic Edition, Harley Davidson, (Stone Mountain, Georgia) 2006.

Honda Civic 2008, CR-V, Kelly Blue Book, Specifications.

Hooker, Brian, et al., "Methodological Issues and Evidence of Malfeasance in Research Purporting to Show Thimerosal in Vaccines Is Safe," BioMed Research International, June 4, 2014, Vol. 2014, Article ID 247218, p. 4-5.

Horne, Tom, email to CDC Diana Schendel, "Application Tech Review," November 13 & 16, 2003.

History Commons: "Context of 'November 2002: US Again Decides Not to Attack Al-Zarqawi Camp in Northern Iraq," History Commons Organization online (Santa Cruz, California).

Huffington, Arianna, "Expect no Patent Law revision in Eli Lilly's Washington," The Islet Foundation online forum, December 4, 2002, posted by Dennis, (United States) August 7, 2003.

International Epidemiology Association, "Past Presidents," (Raleigh, North Carolina): http://ieaweb.org/about-iea/history/past-presidents/.

Jørgensen, Jørgen, "Aarhus University Statement on Dr. Poul Thorsen," January 22, 2010.

King, Martin Luther, Jr., "I have a Dream" Speech, Government Archives, (Washington, DC), 1963.

Le Zotte, Jennifer, "How the Summer of Atomic Bomb Testing Turned the Bikini Into a Phenomenon," Smithsonian.com, Smithsonian Magazine, (Washington, DC) May 21, 2015.

Lehmann, Cristof, "Congressman Blasts CDC for Incestuous Relationship with Vaccine Makers," NSNBC International Online, April 17, 2014.

Lehrer, Jim, "The Anthrax Threat: Dr. Jeffrey Koplan, Director of the CDC," PBS News Hour with Jim Lehrer, (New York, NY) October 24, 2001.

List of Nobel Laureates, Denmark, Wikileaks.org, (Copenhagen, Denmark) April 2012.

Luther, Linda G., *"Mercury Products and Waste: Legislative and Regulatory Activities to Control Mercury,"* Environmental Policy Analyst, Resources, Science, and Industry Division, Wikileaks.org (Stockholm, Sweden), May 12, 2003, pp. 2, 9-11.

Madsen, Kreesten M, email to James O. Grundvig, "12 Questions for Interview," (Copenhagen, Denmark) June 27, 2015.

Madsen, Kreesten Meldgaard, LinkedIn.com profile.

*Marshall Islands Moment,* Editorial: The New York Sun, (New York, New York) April

Maugh, Thomas H. II, "Obituary: Maurice R. Hilleman, 85; Scientist Developed Many

Vaccines That Saved Millions of Lives," Los Angeles Times, (Los Angeles), April 13, 2005.

Mcauley, Erin, "Dad Pushing Autism Link Can Get More from CDC," Courthouse News Service, (Pasadena, California) August 24, 2012, p. 1.

McClam, Erin, "CDC Chief Jeffrey Koplon Resigns," Associated Press, (New York, NY) February 2, 2002.

Mendability Organization, "Our Brains and Metals," Sensory Enrichment Therapy (Irvine, California), 2011. http://www.mendability.com/articles/our-brain-and-metals/

Miller, Zeke J., "Obama Appoints Ron Klain as Ebola Czar," Time Magazine, (New York, NY) October 17, 2014.

Moyers, Bill, "Troubled Waters," NOW with Bill Moyers, NPR, December 20, 2002.

*NANEA-CDC Cooperative Agreement, Budget: Year 3, Feb 2004-Jan 2005,* Centers for Disease Control, provided by Dr. Brian Hooker's 2004 FOIA request (Atlanta, Georgia) December 6, 2003, p. 2.

National Center for Birth Defects and Developmental Disabilities, Centers for Disease Control "Timeline – 2001" (Atlanta, Georgia). http://www.cdc.gov/ncbddd/aboutus/timeline/timeline-interactive.html

Naumann, Rebecca B., and Bethany A. West, "Motor Vehicle—Related Deaths—United States, 2003-2007," Morbidity and Mortality Weekly Report, National Center for Injury Prevention and Control, CDC (Atlanta, Georgia), January 14, 2011, 60(01);52-55

Obituary: "Obituary of Diana Ruth Wise Schendel," The Times and Democrat, (Columbia, South Carolina), May 08, 2008. October 12, 2008.

Olivarius, NF, et al. "The Danish National Health Service Register. A tool for primary health care research," Danish Medical Bulletin, 1997 Sept. 44(4):44953.

Olsen, Jørn, "Biography: Jørn Olsen," Southern California Injury Research Program, UCLA School of Public Health (Los Angeles, California):

Olsen, Jørn, EpiBlog, "Conflicts of Interest," International Epidemiology Association, (Aarhus, Denmark) February 12, 2014.

*Operation Ranch Hand,* Wikipedia.org (United States), December 2008.

Østjllands Police: "Anklageskrift Domsmandssag—'tax indictment'— Poul Thorsen," East Jutland Police, Court Report, (Aarhus, Denmark) March 16, 2009.

Parner, Erik, et al., "Autism Prevalence Trends Over Time in Denmark," JAMA ArchPeciatrics.com, (Chicago, Illinois), December 2008;162(12):1150-1156.

Ramirez, Alvaro, Deck: "European Autism Information System," EAIS-Project Alvaro Ramirez (looking a lot like Martin Knapp) 2008, slides 15-17.

Ramskov, Jens, "Controversial Danish Researcher Released of Punitive Tax in Related Fraud," Ingeniøren: Engineering Magazine, (Copenhagen, Denmark) March 27, 2012.

Richter Lise, "Danish Researcher in Consumption Trap," Information. DK, (Copenhagen, Denmark), May 23, 2011, pp. 3-4.

Roberts, Joel, "The Man Behind the Vaccine Mystery," CBS Evening News, December 12, 2002.

Rohde, Wayne, "The Vaccine Court: The Dark Truth of America's Vaccine Injury Compensation Program," Skyhorse Publishing, (New York, NY) 2014, p. 5 & 149.

Ross, Robert, "Julie Gerberding Names Director of CDC," CIDRAP News (Center for Infectious Disease Research and Policy), University of Minnesota, (Minneapolis, Minnesota), July 3, 2002.

Schendel, Diana E., "Biography: Diana Schendel," Dept. of Public Health, Aarhus University (Aarhus, Denmark), 2014.

Schendel, Diana E., Dept. of Health, Aarhus University, to James O. Grundvig, "Poul Thorsen," (Aarhus, Denmark), July 3, 2015.

Schendel, Diana E., Epidemiology Research Scientist, Dept. of Health, Aarhus University, email to James O. Grundvig, "Poul Thorsen" (Aarhus, Denmark) July 3, 2015.

Schendel, Diana, Centers for Disease Control Application Affidavit for Employment, (Atlanta, Georgia) November 1992.

Schendel, Diana, Centers for Disease Control Appointment Affidavits, (Atlanta, Georgia) April 19, 1993.

Simpson, Diane, email to Bob Chen, "UK Vaccine Schedule and Thimerosal Exposure," Centers for Disease Control, (Atlanta, Georgia), June 25, 2001.

Simpson, Diane, email to Christopher Gillberg, "Autism Data in Sweden," Centers for Disease Control, (Atlanta, Georgia), August 7, 2001.

Simpson, Diane, email to Jeanette and Paul Stehr-Green, "Ongoing Investigation of

Thimerosal," Centers for Disease Control, (Atlanta, Georgia), August 6, 2001.

Simpson, Diane, email to Kreesten M. Madsen, University of Aarhus, Dept. of Epidemiology, Aarhus, Denmark, "Autism Data" Centers for Disease Control, (Atlanta, Georgia), June 12, 2001.

Simpson, Diane, email to Marta Granstrom, Medical Products Agency, Uppsala, Sweden, "Vaccine Preservatives" Centers for Disease Control, (Atlanta, Georgia) June 11, 2001.

Simpson, Diane, email to Poul Thorsen, NANEA, Aarhus, Denmark, "Charts," Centers for Disease Control, (Atlanta, Georgia), August 2, 2001.

Simpson, Diane, email to Marshalyn Yeargin-Allsopp, "Data from Denmark," Centers for Disease Control, (Atlanta, Georgia) June 8, 2001.

Skou, Jens Christian, Wikileaks.org, (Copenhagen, Denmark) February 2013.

Sodium-Potassium Adenosine Triphosphatase, Wikileaks.org, (United States) January 27, 2016. https://en.wikipedia.org/wiki/Na%2B/K%2B-ATPase.

Sovereign Wealth Fund Index: http://www.swfinstitute.org/fund-rankings/.

Steenhuysen, Julie, "CDC says Flu Shots may not be Good Match for 2014-15 Virus," Reuters, (New York, NY) December 3, 2014.

Stehr-Greene, Paul, email to Diane Simpson, "Ongoing Investigation of Thimerosal," Centers for Disease Control, (Atlanta, Georgia), August 6, 2001.

Stephenson, PhD, Joan, "New IOM Report Links Agent Orange Exposure to Risk of Birth Defect in Vietnam Vets' Children,"

*JAMA* (Chicago, Illinois), April 10, 1996, Vol. 275, No. 14, pp. 1066-1067.

*The Agent Orange Record Map,* Agent Orange Record, (Chester, Vermont): www.agentorangerecord.com/information/what_is_dioxin/sites/

Thompson, William W., "Press Release Statement of William W. Thompson Regarding 2004 Article Examining the Possibility of a Relationship Between MMR Vaccines and Autism," Morgan Verkamp LLC, (Cincinnati, Ohio) August 27, 2014.

Thorsen, Niels B., Gravestone at Grinderslev Church, (Roslev, Denmark), 1984.

Thorsen, Poul, "Curriculum Vitae: Poul Thorsen," Drexel University, (Philadelphia, Pennsylvania) January 22, 2010.

Thorsen, Poul, "Home Renter," Personer.Eniro.SE (Stocksund, Sweden) 2012.

Thorsen, Poul, et al., "Identification of Biological/Biochemical Marker(s) for Preterm Delivery," Blackwell Science, Ltd., Paediatric and Perinatal Epidemiology, (Aarhus, Denmark) 2001 (Suppl. 2), p. 90-103.

Thorsen, Poul, et. al., Reply to Letter to Editor: "Sensitivity of ligase chain reaction assay of urine from pregnant women for Chlamydiatrachomatis," *The Lancet,* (London, UK) April 5, 1997.

Thorsen, Poul, Managing Director, NANEA, Aarhus University, to Brian Hooker, "Role at the CDC," (Aarhus, Denmark) November 24, 2004.

*Three Canadian Soldiers Sick with Superbug,* UPI, August 20, 2009.

Thrower, David email to James O. Grundvig, (United Kingdom) July 13, 2015.

Toner, Mike, "U.S. Like Sent Iraq Toxic Bugs," Atlanta-Journal Constitution, (Atlanta, Georgia) October 2, 2002.

*Tourists Flock to Witness Fall of Wall Street,* Europe Turbo News, (New York, NY) October 13, 2008.

Truman, Harry S., "Truman Bomb Test: General Leslie Groves describes a weapon of mass destruction—War Department, Memorandum for the Secretary of War," General Leslie Groves, *American Experience*, PBS.org, (Washington, DC) July 18, 1945.

University of Aarhus Press Release: *Jørgen Jørgensen is the Director of the University of Aarhus.* Dagens Medicin, February 24, 2009.

Vancouver Protocol, the Fifth Addition (1997), p. 1.

Verstraeten, Thomas, email to Bob Davis: "It Just Won't Go Away," Centers for Disease Control, (Atlanta, Georgia) December 17, 1999.

Verstraeten, Thomas, email to Philippe Grandjean, "Thimerosal and Neurologic Outcomes," Centers for Disease Control, (Atlanta, Georgia), July 14, 2000.

Viking Ship Museum, Roskilde, Wikipedia.com, (Roskilde, Denmark), modified on January 9, 2016.

Vogel, Ida, Dept. of Health, Aarhus University Hospital, email to James O. Grundvig, "Poul Thorsen," (Aarhus, Denmark) June 2, 2015.

Wayback Time Machine, NANEA Team (Aarhus, Denmark): http://web.archive.org/web/20021215062608/http:/www.nanea.dk/team/team_aarhus.html

Wikipedia, Bright Collaboration: https://en.wikipedia.org/wiki/Brighton_Collaboration.

Yates, Sally Quillian, U.S. District Attorney, Dept. of Justice, "U.S. vs. Poul Thorsen," Case 1:11-cr-00194-UNA, Doc 1, (Atlanta, Georgia) Filed April 13, 2011, pp. 1, 6, 8.

Yeargin-Allsopp, Marshalyn email to Jose Cordero, "Proposal for Study of MMR Vaccine and Autism in Denmark," Centers for Disease Control, (Atlanta, Georgia) May 30, 2001.

Zumwalt Admiral Elmo R., "Declassified Testimony before 101st Congress," (Washington, DC), May 5, 1990.

*Interviews:*

The author conducted more than a dozen interviews with key people for the story, including but not limited to, Kreesten M. Madsen (Copenhagen, Denmark); Palle Valentiner-Branth, Statens Serum Institut (Copenhagen, Denmark); Fleming Svith, Dept. of Journalism, Aarhus University (Aarhus, Denmark); Dr. Brian Hooker (California); Mark Blaxill (Boston, Massachusetts); Dr. F. Edward Yazbak (Falmouth, Massachusetts); Robert Krakow, Esq. (New York, NY); John Stone (London, UK); several Danish journalists and private investigators.

# ABOUT THE AUTHOR

**James Ottar Grundvig** is a first generation Norwegian–American and father of a teenage autistic son, who is learning how to speak for the first time after years of medical intervention, including Transcranial Direct Current Stimulation therapy under the guidance of Dr. Harry Schneider in a Columbia University chartered study, from 2009–2014.

Mr. Grundvig has spent thirty years of his professional career in the engineering–construction space, working on projects of scale in Norway, Philadelphia, New Jersey, and New York City. For the past dozen years, he took his project management research skills and applied them to his son's mental health crises and began to write the five-year-old boy's journey in 2005 with the *Epoch Times*. This decade, he has published a broad array of health, technology, and environmental subjects in the *Huffington Post, Financial Times Foreign Direct Investment Magazine, Law.com, and Autism Spectrum News*, among other media outlets.

Mr. Grundvig has two other books with Skyhorse Publishing coming to the market: *Breaking Van Gogh: Saint-Rémy, Forgery, and the $95 Million Fake at the Met*, and a techno thriller novel, *Dolphin Drone*.